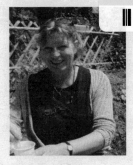

Maggie Groff is a multi-award-winning novelist, columnist and non-fiction writer living and working in Australia. As a young woman in England she trained as a state registered nurse at King's College Hospital, London, before pursuing a richly varied nursing career, much of it at iconic locations. Aware that her daughter knew little about her professional life prior to becoming an author, she was inspired to write this nursing memoir.

Maggie's previous books include the bestselling *Mothers Behaving Badly* which showcased her hilarious experiences as a mother, *Hoax Cuisine* which recounted her domestic dramas in the kitchen, and the highly-acclaimed crime novels featuring investigative journalist Scout Davis: *Mad Men, Bad Girls*, and *Good News, Bad News*, voted in 2013 as one of the top fifty books you can't put down.

www.penguin.co.uk

MAGGIE GROFF

Not Your Average Nurse

The Entertaining True Story of a Student Nurse in 1970s London

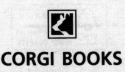

CORGI BOOKS

TRANSWORLD PUBLISHERS
61–63 Uxbridge Road, London W5 5SA
www.penguin.co.uk

Transworld is part of the Penguin Random House group of companies
whose addresses can be found at global.penguinrandomhouse.com

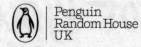

Penguin
Random House
UK

First published in Great Britain in 2017 by Corgi Books
an imprint of Transworld Publishers

This book is a work of non-fiction based on the life, experiences and
recollections of the author. In some limited cases names of people, places,
dates, sequences or the detail of events have been changed solely to protect
the privacy of others. The author has stated to the publishers that,
except in such minor respects not affecting the substantial
accuracy of the work, the contents of this book are true.

Every effort has been made to obtain the necessary permissions with
reference to copyright material, both illustrative and quoted. We apologize
for any omissions in this respect and will be pleased to make the
appropriate acknowledgements in any future edition.

A CIP catalogue record for this book
is available from the British Library.

ISBN
9780552174145

Typeset in 11.75/13.75pt Berkeley by Jouve (UK), Milton Keynes.
Printed and bound in Great Britain by Clays Ltd, Bungay, Suffolk.

Penguin Random House is committed to a sustainable
future for our business, our readers and our planet. This book
is made from Forest Stewardship Council® certified paper.

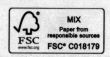

MIX
Paper from
responsible sources
FSC
www.fsc.org   FSC® C018179

1 3 5 7 9 10 8 6 4 2

Author's Note

Although I didn't realize it at the time, I was fortunate to train at London's King's College Hospital, one of the largest and busiest teaching hospitals in Britain. Somehow, King's took a rather selfish and opinionated girl and moulded her into a halfway decent human being and, I like to think, a first-rate nurse. Truly, there is something about the place that seeps into your bones.

Everything written here really happened. Apart from my family, nearly all the names have been changed to protect identities. Some of my friends appear as themselves, and are happy to do so. Others have been merged to avoid confusion. For obvious privacy reasons, I have also altered details concerning the timing of incidents and the place where they happened, and I have consolidated some events to better tell the story. As you do.

Contents

CONTENTS

CHAPTER 1

Fox Hunting for Beginners

A teaching hospital in London: September 1970

BIG TROUBLE AWAITED me on my first day on the job, but I wasn't a bit surprised. The god of bright young things has always had a custard tart ready to smack in the face of a girl like me.

Green as a spring twig, I'd completed two weeks of basic nursing instruction in a classroom and was spending a supervised morning on a ward, one of several such half-days that would occur before the end of two months' Preliminary Training School (PTS), if I lasted that long.

'You elderly men need to look neat and tidy,' I told Mr Snape, as I straightened his top sheet.

'Oh, go away, you stupid girl,' he snarled. 'I've got socks older than you!' Sticking out a determined chin, he messed up the sheet and childishly kicked his legs about.

Challenged, I threw him the death stare I'd perfected in 1957 in the playground at Castle Street Primary School. In return, Snape launched his version of the same look he had perfected in 1916 in the war-torn trenches of the Western Front. Back and forth our faces raged until, totally outclassed, I turned away.

To the casual observer, I was a fresh-faced eighteen-year-old girl, dressed in a newly minted King's College Hospital student-nurse uniform. My crown was a paper cap attached to my strawberry-blonde up-do with hairgrips, and my overly long blue-and-white-striped waisted dress was protected from germ warfare by a starched white apron that could stand up on its own.

From my perspective, I looked fabulous – very cool and now – and the only problem with the image was that I wasn't actually at King's College Hospital. Somehow a terrible mistake had occurred, and I was standing in what appeared to be a dilapidated eighteenth-century school hall, but was in reality a male geriatric ward at St Giles Hospital in Camberwell, an area of South London classified as a Poor Law parish in 1835. And not much had changed.

Formerly a workhouse for the destitute, St Giles had been developed into an infirmary about a hundred years before I arrived, and its present state of crumbling antiquity was three moons and a shooting star away from the grandeur and excitement of King's College Hospital in Denmark Hill, where I was supposed to be. I planned on writing a stern letter when I discovered who was responsible for this appalling mix-up.

Around me on the ward, which was unimaginatively identified by a capital letter and a number, and which I am rechristening 'Dickens', courtesy of the workhouse connection, the air was filled with groans, vocal complaints, death-rattling coughs and unpleasant odours.

Scurrying about in this oppressive atmosphere,

second- and third-year student nurses delivered bowls of steaming water, pulled curtains around beds, lifted men on to wheelchairs and pushed them here and there, filled things, emptied things, and wrestled with trolleys and oxygen cylinders. Frustrated that a staff nurse had directed me to pointlessly tidy top sheets, I observed the other nurses' purposeful industry with mounting annoyance.

Another new student nurse, Fenella, was also on Dickens. A tall, dark-haired girl with lovely apple cheeks and a plummy voice, Fenella wouldn't have been out of place on a hockey field at an English boarding school. On arrival, she was dispatched to the clinical room to clean lotion cupboards, and I was pleased it was her, not me: I would have broken a bottle of rare potion from the Amazon that had cost a hundred pounds. I was safer with sheets. It's pretty hard to break sheets.

I was straightening the bedding of a sleeping man when a cross-looking woman in a green sister's uniform marched on to the ward and headed towards me. Short and scrawny, with a malignant fierceness behind her steel-grey eyes, she was identified by her name badge as Sister Morag, the ward sister who was to supervise me.

'Good morning, Sister,' I said, with the confidence of someone who has practised the line while watching *Dr Finlay's Casebook* on TV. Surely now I would be allocated a sensible job.

Sister Morag frowned. Uh-oh . . . maybe she thought this sheet-tidying lark was my idea.

'Staff Nurse told me to tidy sheets,' I said accusingly, and scoffed for good measure.

'It's important for beds to look tidy,' she said sharply.

'And when you've finished that, you are to disinfect everything in the sluice, scrub the bath and bowls in the bathroom, wash the tooth mugs and spittoons, clean the flower vases, wet-dust the patients' bedside lockers and then prepare the kitchen trolley for the patients' morning tea.'

Hmm? That didn't sound right. Shouldn't I be bed-bathing patients and taking temperatures? Practising things I had learned in class? Nothing she mentioned required supervision or special instruction. I mean, I already knew how to clean. Who didn't?

Genuinely puzzled, I asked, 'Is it the cleaner's day off?'

Wrong question, Maggie. Sister Morag narrowed her eyes and pressed her thin, bloodless lips together. Thrusting out a furious pointy finger, she ordered, 'Get to work!'

Now, here's the thing: I was already standing where I needed to be, so what was I supposed to do? Thankfully, flight mode kicked in and I walked swiftly away. And I kept walking until Sister Morag disappeared into her office to breakfast on bullets and eye of newt.

Left to supervise myself, and scared that every patient might have a heart attack, I cautiously approached the nearest bed. Cleverly, I checked the patient's name on the label clipped to the iron bed-head. Plaques identifying the consultants' names were displayed above the beds. Like religious icons.

'How are you, Mr Cartwright?' I asked brightly, as I straightened his sheet.

'What's it to you?' he grumbled.

'S-sorry,' I stammered. 'Can I get you anything?'

4

'A cure would be good,' he replied, and I laughed because I thought it was funny.

'That wasn't a joke,' he said indignantly. 'Now go and annoy somebody else.'

As I moved from bed to bed, a pattern was emerging: politeness from me, rudeness from patients.

'Good morning, Mr Pettigrew,' I said.

'What's good about it?' he wheezed.

'Can I straighten your sheet, Mr Hogg?'

'No! Sod off!'

Disheartened, I surveyed the human landscape. There were twenty-four men slumped in beds and armchairs around the ward, and all of them were older than God with forests growing out of their ears. Victims of strokes, dicky tickers, pneumonia, liver disease and other failing organs, I tried to normalize the men by telling myself that each of them was someone's grandfather – a dear old soul with a favourite cap and an unfinished wood project in his shed – but the idea didn't work. They were simply too horrid.

'Are all elderly male patients unpleasant?' I asked an attractive student nurse, Rosie O'Brien, when our paths crossed at the wall sink halfway down the ward.

'Only those on Dickens,' she said, and tucked loose strands of Titian hair under her second-year frilly hat. 'But it's nothing an AK-47 wouldn't fix.'

My laughter drew Sister Morag's attention. Through the glass in her office window, she fixed me with an icy stare that seemed to be saying, 'You are enjoying yourself and it has to stop.'

'Whoops,' Rosie said, and I grimaced. I liked Rosie instantly. Where other nurses bustled about, Rosie appeared to glide everywhere like a swan. I was pleased when we were sent to morning tea together in the hospital refectory.

'We really shouldn't judge the patients harshly,' Rosie advised me. 'You have to remember that most of them are poorly educated, working-class men who've had their lives torn apart by war, injury and the Depression.'

That pretty much defined my mother's father, Grandpa Leonard Higgins, and he hadn't been disagreeable. I mentioned this to Rosie.

'I suppose I shouldn't make excuses for them,' she reasoned, then lit a cigarette and blew smoke rings in the air. 'But they've lost their place in the world and I feel sorry for them. I can't help it.'

Impressed by her generous attitude, but far from understanding it, I asked, 'Are they rude to Sister Morag and the doctors?'

Rosie shook her head. 'Good Lord, no, Maggie. They resent us because we're young, independent girls pursuing a career. To them, we should be married and having babies. Besides, they know they can be as rude to us as they want.'

'Why is that?' I asked, a smidgen alarmed.

'Because everyone else is,' Rosie quipped, and we laughed, although my mirth was tinged with concern.

Back on the ward, and wary of any conversation that might elicit verbal abuse, I wiped bedside lockers in silence. Once I was satisfied they were in showroom condition, I prepared the tea trolley in the kitchen and wheeled it on to the ward.

'Would you like tea, Mr Tucker?' I asked the first patient.

Fumbling with something under his blanket, he muttered, 'No. Bugger off!'

Averting my eyes, I hastily rolled the trolley forward.

'Would you like a drink, Mr Clegg?' I asked, reading the name from a chart hanging on the end of the bed.

'Scotch and soda,' replied a frail voice. Surprised, I looked properly at Mr Clegg. Dribble and dandruff aside, I could have hugged him. I remembered from the night nurse's report that Mr Clegg had congestive cardiac failure, although I wasn't sure what that was.

'I can only do tea,' I said regretfully.

'Then tea it is,' he replied softly. 'Milk, no sugar, please, love.'

Happy to encounter good manners, I set the tea on the bed-table and helped him sit up.

'Thank you,' he said, his voice stronger once he was upright. 'First day?'

'Yes, until lunchtime.'

'You'll be fine,' he assured me.

'I hope so,' I said, and with great trepidation I pushed the trolley to the end of Mr Snape's bed.

'Tea?' I offered nervously.

'Milk, two sugars,' he said curtly.

Trembling, I placed the tea on his bedside locker. I hadn't stirred the sugar and I didn't leave a teaspoon. On purpose, I think.

Moving along, I sublimated my angst with an enforced sunny disposition and completed the tea round as quickly as possible. As I pushed the trolley back past Mr Clegg, he beckoned me over. 'Don't mind old Snape, love,' he whispered. 'He's had Hong Kong flu and now he has bronchitis. He was a prisoner of war and he got the cholera. And his wife is dead. That doesn't do much for his sense of humour.'

Seized by guilt, I took Mr Snape a teaspoon and asked whether he had fought in the First World War or the Second World War. Maybe if I showed an interest, it might improve his demeanour.

Big mistake, Maggie. Big. Mr Snape struggled to sit up, an activity that caused a world-class coughing fit. Uncertain what to do, I returned to the tea trolley and hid from view by crouching down as if I had important business on the lower shelf. With the biscuits. The ones I had forgotten to serve.

Oh, what the heck? I thought, and while I was down there I popped one of the tempting chocolate Digestives into my mouth. What can I say? There they were, and there I was . . .

'Johnson! What do you think you're doing?' barked an angry voice. I looked up to see Sister Morag, her face flushed scarlet and on the point of explosion.

Trying to swallow a mouthful, I mumbled, 'I'm sowee, Sister Mawag.'

Huffing loudly, she ordered a passing nurse to help Mr Snape. As her angry footsteps marched away, I could hear her sarcastically chanting, 'So-wee, so-wee, so-wee . . .'

'I expect she's gone to get her elephant gun,' Mr Clegg said, but I was too ashamed to laugh.

When Mr Snape had recovered, and most of his lungs were on the far wall, he managed to croak hoarsely at me, 'It was the *Great War*, you bleedin' idiot!'

That did it! I'd had a snoot-full of vulgar men and I snapped. Hands on hips and head tilted, I said cockily, 'I think you'll find that these days we call it the First World War.'

8

Mr Snape turned red to the roots of his hair and the veins in his neck stood out like ropes. It looked as if his head was going to launch clean off his shoulders. Unbelievable, really, causing two exploding heads on my first day. It had to be some sort of student-nurse record.

Leaning forward, Snape fixed me in his crosshairs. 'Soldiers who served in the Great War,' he roared angrily, 'call it the *Great War!*' He took a big gulp of air and added menacingly, 'We didn't know there was going to be a Second World War, did we?'

Ouch! In my naivety, I hadn't yet learned that the hunter harpoons the whale when she surfaces to blow. Snape had shot me right between the eyes, and all I could do was gush, 'I'm so dreadfully sorry.'

The cavalry, in the form of Mr Clegg, came to my rescue. 'That's interesting, Snape,' he said, his tone measured. 'I've never thought of it like that before.'

Mr Snape flopped back on to his pillows, closed his eyes and swore prodigiously. Mildly panicked, I looked around to see whether Sister Morag had heard the goings-on. Luckily, she was nowhere in sight – probably lying down with a cold compress on her forehead.

'Oh dear, I can't seem to do anything right,' I said to Mr Clegg.

'Never mind, love,' he replied, and managed a weak smile. A little short of breath, he turned his oxygen on and held the mask over his face.

Despondent, I went to re-clean the tooth mugs and spittoons, almost knocking myself out with disinfectant fumes. After a while, my good husbandry was interrupted by a plump staff nurse. Only a few years my senior, she said, 'Johnson, go and bed-bath Mr Gribble in bed four.'

'Righty-ho,' I chirped. Finally some real nursing.

' "Yes, Staff Nurse" will do, Johnson,' she replied tersely.

What was wrong with these people? Ticked off, I christened her Staff Nurse Tubby.

Along with fifty-seven other girls in my set, I had watched our nurse tutor, a pleasant-looking woman called Sister Bronwyn, demonstrate on a dummy in the classroom how to bed-bath a bedridden patient with a bar of Lifebuoy, a flannel and two towels. Her method was efficient, practical and clinical; sentiment and leisurely pampering, she assured us, were for idealistic time-wasters. It would be a while before I learned of the comfort and solace that the warm, gentle touch of a caring nurse could bring to the sick, the wounded, the old and the frightened.

Unfortunately it looked like I would be bed-bathing Mr Gribble alone. Rosie had gone to help on another ward, Fenella was busy restocking shelves, and I couldn't find anyone free to help me. So much, I thought, for supervision.

To put Mr Gribble at ease, I acted as though I had performed a million bed-baths. Outwardly confident, I fetched a bowl of hot water from the bathroom and placed it on Mr Gribble's bed-table. Inwardly, I was shaking. At morning report, I had learned that Mr Gribble was eighty-four and had something called Graves' disease. Assuming it would shortly be game over for old Gribble, it was with appropriate solemnity that I set about making his last moments on earth more comfortable. *Oh well, here goes*, I told myself.

Gingerly, I closed the curtains around his bed.

'I am going to give you a bed-bath, Mr Gribble,' I said, my voice vaguely tremulous.

Mr Gribble had large, staring eyes and appeared jolly pleased at the news. Enthusiastically, he undid the rubber buttons on his National Health pyjamas. Taking care, I helped him remove his pyjama top.

'Good grief!' I blurted out, as a magnificent tattoo revealed itself. Covering Mr Gribble's chest, arms and back – in fact, every spare inch of skin – was an intricately drawn scene of a fox hunt, with horses and riders, bugles and hounds.

'Pretty good, eh?' he said, holding out his arms and proudly surveying his body.

'I'll say,' I said. It was the first tattoo I had ever seen.

'You should see where the fox is hiding!' he said, and before I could stop him Mr Gribble flipped on to his side and pulled down his pyjama pants.

I gasped in amazement. The foxhounds, their eyes blazing and their tongues hanging out, were racing across Mr Gribble's bottom towards his anus, emerging from which was the splendid plume of a fox tail.

A blush spread across my skin, and I busied myself with organizing towels, flannel and soap. Starting at the top and in silence, because I had no idea what to say, I washed Mr Gribble's face and dried it. It would have taken a machete to penetrate his nose hair, so I gave his nostrils a wide berth.

Standing back, I looked at him. So far so good. He was still alive.

As gently as if I were icing a wedding cake, and fascinated by the tattoo, I washed his arms and chest, then dried them. Without my having to ask, Mr Gribble sat forward and I washed his back. During all this soap and water anointing, it had not escaped my attention that there were frequent outbursts of laughter from the other side of the curtains.

Hang on a minute.

Patients who needed a bed-bath were critically ill, incapacitated and incapable of washing themselves. That was the whole point of it. Mr Gribble was as agile as a cat . . .

Oh, marvellous! This was one of those new-girl tricks, like being sent downstairs for a long weight (a long wait). Or to the stores for a fallopian tube.

'I've been had, haven't I?' I said glumly, and bit my lip.

Mr Gribble nodded. 'Never mind, ducks. Better me than those other grumpy bastards.'

Conceding he had a point, I asked hopefully, 'You haven't really got Graves' disease, have you?' I had taken quite a shine to Alf Gribble.

'Oh, yes,' he said. 'But I'm not for the knacker's yard. It's named after a Paddy doctor called Graves. I'm producing too much thyroid hormone. The medical ward I'm supposed to be on is full, but there should be a bed soon.' Medical wards, Rosie had told me, were where patients had their illness treated with medications, physiotherapy and bed rest.

'That's good,' I said, pleased he wasn't dying. And then, always up for a bit of revenge, I had an idea. 'Will you stay in bed? Behind the curtains?' I asked eagerly.

'Anything, ducks,' he replied. 'I owe you one.'

Adopting an anxious face, I exited the curtains and hurried towards Sister Morag's office. Hearing loud sniggers, I turned my head and saw Staff Nurse

Tubby and a patient quickly look away. My discomfort was apparently high entertainment.

'Sister Morag!' I cried, feigning panic as I entered the office, where she and two other ward sisters were rushed off their feet drinking tea. 'There's been an accident. The soap I used has made the ink run on Mr Gribble's tattoo!'

'What?' Sister Morag exclaimed. Her face drained of colour and she stood up. 'What did you say, Johnson?'

'Oh, what have I done?' I wailed.

There was a mass exodus as the sisters bolted from the office and raced to Mr Gribble's bedside. Hastily, I made my escape to a nearby churchyard and sat on the damp grass and cried, but not because I was so easily duped. Or because I'd just learned that Jimi Hendrix had died.

No. The real blow I was coming to grips with was much worse. Fenella had told me that she and I would be spending the next four months of our ward clinical training on Dickens, which meant full time at the end of Preliminary Training School.

How had I not realized this before?

Not paying attention, according to Fenella.

Really, it was too awful for words.

In class, during the afternoon, it became apparent that PTS nurses had been allocated to several different hospitals in the area. Mrs Clemens, from the School of Nursing, asked us to share our ward experiences.

'I loved it,' said one.

'It was everything I'd hoped it would be,' crowed another.

'Well, blow that for a game of raspberries,'

complained a disgruntled voice in the back row, and everyone turned to look at me.

Taken aback that I had voiced my feelings aloud, I stared open-mouthed and wide-eyed at the student nurse sitting next to me as though it was her, not me, who had spoken. A tall, elegant girl with laughing eyes, her name was Jan, and she rested those eyes on my face and beamed the most beguiling smile. Jan knew exactly what I was doing, and in that moment a friendship was born.

Mrs Clemens, acting as though nothing untoward had occurred, chivvied the class for more feedback. In response, girls who had been placed at St Francis, the geriatric hospital in East Dulwich, spoke candidly of their disappointment. Several complained that they had found the work heavy and the physical frailties and incontinence confronting. One admitted she was already thinking of leaving.

This feedback was too honest.

'If you don't want to work hard,' Mrs Clemens warned, 'then you are embarking on the wrong profession.'

In response, the St Francis nurses visibly shrank, and I felt sorry for them, especially when students on exciting wards at King's boasted of watching suture removal and intravenous (IV) infusions being established. Sutures? IV infusions? I listened, green with envy.

Students on general medical and surgical wards at Dulwich Hospital had received instruction in cardiac care and pre- and post-operative care, and had practised bed-bathing and bed-making. However, all was not tickety-boo. One nurse on a surgical ward reported that she'd had no supervision as senior nurses were too busy. Like an infectious yawn, other nurses voiced the same concern. Visibly irritated by this information, Mrs Clemens shot a disapproving look at the nurse who had raised the matter.

When it came to Fenella's turn to share, she smartly reported having spent a good morning on Dickens. The news brought a satisfied smile to Mrs Clemens's face.

'Aren't you on Dickens as well?' Jan asked me, in a hushed voice.

I nodded. 'And it was awful,' I whispered back.

Privately, I wondered whether Fenella and the St Francis nurses had rumbled, as I had, that our geriatric ward allocations were designed to weed out those of us the tutors thought unsuited to nursing. With her mildly superior air and upper-class diction, Fenella was surely a target for their misguided suspicions. I hadn't yet figured out why they thought I might be unsuitable. Maybe because I was.

'And how was *your* morning?' Mrs Clemens asked me, interrupting my thoughts. There wasn't any hint that she knew I was the 'game of raspberries' girl.

In a passable Welsh accent, I said, 'Fantastic, thank you. The old men at St Giles were very nice.'

Jan almost fell off her chair with amusement, and I suppressed a laugh.

The next moment, an office assistant peered round the door and told Mrs Clemens that she had a phone call. Five minutes later, she returned looking rattled.

'Nurses,' she said. 'I have received disturbing news. One of you advised a patient that his wife could bring their dog to the ward during visiting hours this afternoon. Fortunately, the animal was intercepted before it entered the ward.'

Everyone looked around to witness the evildoer behind this dastardly crime, but no one owned up. There were murmurs about infection, dog bites, distemper, and how could anyone be so stupid. I didn't think it was at all stupid because Mr Clegg had asked me so nicely – and he'd been one of only two pleasant patients: he and Mr Gribble, the fox-hunting man.

Avoiding eye contact with Mrs Clemens, I was relieved when she went on to outline future subjects: admission procedures, nursing infectious patients, pain medication, intramuscular injections, operating the autoclave (to sterilize instruments) and care of pressure areas.

'Any questions?' she asked.

'When will our clipboards be issued?' asked a breathless blonde with big blue eyes. Her name was Tilly and she was wearing coral-pink lipstick – a daring offence that scored highly on my friendship-selection criteria. Wearing make-up was strictly forbidden.

'What clipboards?' Mrs Clemens enquired.

'The ones that nurses carry on television,' Tilly explained.

Mrs Clemens appeared confused, but I knew what Tilly meant. Anyone who watched TV hospital dramas would think that nurses spent all day walking around with clipboards. Occasionally they made notes on the clipboards. Mostly, though, they put down the clipboards and kissed a doctor.

Mrs Clemens didn't make the connection, but many of us did. Realizing that Tilly was playing the dumb-blonde card for a laugh, I rewarded her effort with a nod of amused admiration, and Tilly returned a winning grin. Kajung! Another friendship was born.

'I don't know what you're talking about,' Mrs Clemens said dismissively. Then she seemed to have an epiphany, while looking at Tilly, and reminded us that marriage was not allowed if we wished to continue our training.

Those of us in the know cast amused eyes towards Adele, a petite, fine-boned brunette with an intelligent face, whose husband, Fraser, was sharing Adele's bed at our nurses' home. Adele was studiously making notes, but her ears were hotly turning red.

Mrs Clemens was on a roll. There was to be no eating on wards, no chatting with patients, no sitting on hospital beds, no talking to doctors (but sleeping with them, Tilly later advised us, was absolutely fine), no nail polish, no chewing gum . . .

My to-do list was running off the page.

At the end of class, Mrs Clemens announced, 'Nurse Johnson, please stay behind.' Her tone, it must be said, was not encouraging.

Oh dear. This could be about the cleaner's day off, the biscuits or the dog – or the tattoo, the First World War, or the sodding raspberries . . .

My money was on the dog.

But then a voice piped up. 'Certainly, Mrs Clemens.'

Huh? Another Nurse Johnson? What luck!

Cowardly secreting myself among the nurses leaving the classroom, I left the other girl to deny all knowledge of my misdeeds, knowing it would soon become clear to Mrs Clemens that she had the wrong Nurse Johnson. By then, of course, I would be halfway to Nova Scotia. But I felt bad about Mr Clegg. He would have been disappointed not to see his beloved Monty, and I vowed to make it up to him.

In the back of my mind, something was telling me to leave this matter alone but, as always, I didn't listen.

In the warm, drowsy stillness of the early evening, I sat on a tree stump in the back garden of our nurses' home, Hambledon House, and viewed the day's events from afar. I lit a Sobranie Black Russian, smoked a little, and gazed over the velvety-green fairways of the ritzy golf course that occupied the land behind us. A grey squirrel ran in short bursts across the grass, stopping to look around, wary of predators.

Suddenly my solitude was interrupted by a nurse frantically calling my name. Stubbing out the cigarette, I climbed back through the open sash window into the house to find out what the fuss was about.

'It's the Queen Mother on the phone,' the nurse puffed, 'calling you from Balmoral Castle.'

Knowing it was my own mother on the phone, I rolled my eyes. Mum believed that embarrassing her children was an art form, and she was very good at it, too.

Thanking the nurse, I calmly made my way to the public phone in the entry hall and picked up the receiver. Several pairs of eyes were watching me.

'Hello, Your Majesty,' I said, and waved my audience away. Reluctantly, they drifted off.

'How was your first day on the ward, darling?' Mum asked. 'Was it full of frightfully old codgers?'

'No,' I lied.

'I bet they made you clean things.'

'Actually, I gave a patient a bed-bath.'

'Oh! Didn't they make you scrub baths and floors? And bottoms?'

'No.'

'Well, they will,' my mother stated confidently. 'To them, you're just a glorified cleaner, mark my words.'

'Don't worry, Mum.'

'Are you smoking?' she asked suspiciously.

'Of course not!'

'And you're not drinking too much alcohol, are you?'

'Don't be silly!'

'I'll pick you up at the railway station if you want to come home,' she suggested hopefully.

'I'm fine, Mum. Honestly.'

But I wasn't fine. Returning outside, I flicked a bug off the tree stump, sat down, and reluctantly admitted that nursing was not what I had expected. Instead of learning about diseases and caring for the sick and injured in the cut and thrust of a modern hospital, I was stuck in an old workhouse with a ward sister who was Mother Teresa's evil twin. On top of that, I was being abused by old men who were the end product of two wars, chronic illness and dispiriting poverty, and all I had done was clean things they might use.

Worse still, there was no one to blame but myself. If I'd read the information provided by King's more closely, I would have realized there were hidden catches in their enticing marketing campaign, the most notable of which was that *the exceptional clinical nurse training* offered by King's College Hospital might not actually be *at* King's College Hospital.

I lit another Sobranie and practised blowing smoke rings, like Rosie O'Brien. Out on the sixteenth fairway, a late golfer was striding towards the green, muttering furiously to himself. Feeling a chill, I pulled my cardigan around my shoulders.

A girl's voice broke the evening air. 'Tilly and I are off to the Crown and Greyhound in Dulwich Village,' Jan yelled through the open window. 'Are you coming, Maggie?'

'I'll be right there,' I called over my shoulder.

To tell you the truth, I was pretty sure this nursing lark wasn't the job for me. But London, though . . . London was bloody marvellous.

CHAPTER 2

London Calling

Merry England: 1952–70

I NEVER WANTED to be a nurse. Not even when my brother Richard and I were children and we removed Johnny Cook's appendix in the air-raid shelter in our back garden. Richard was the surgeon general, Mr Sawbones, and I was the anaesthetist, Miss Fifi de la Bon Bon. Johnny was always the patient and his made-up name was always Johnny Cook.

Fast-forward a dozen or so years and the idea of nursing still hadn't crossed my mind. Nor was I remotely cut from the traditional 'angel-of-mercy' cloth. According to Richard, I was fashioned from a more 'know-it-all' type of material, which was quite true and proved to be a tremendous stroke of luck. You see, if I hadn't been a self-absorbed, single-minded teenager hell-bent on moving to London, I would never have become a nurse at all.

For as long as for ever, I had wanted to be a writer, but as the 1960s swung into the 1970s, the general consensus at sherry parties in Fareham, the coastal market town near Portsmouth we had moved to when I was ten, was that writing offered limited prospects of success for a woman and therefore no financial security. The other objection – the one expressed with greater concern – was the unlikely prospect of meeting a suitable husband.

'She'll never find a man, Marion,' a neighbour told my mother. 'Not with a solitary job like writing.'

'Maggie will be on the shelf, and that's a fact,' said our daily cleaner, Mrs Preston, a world authority on varicose veins and *Coronation Street*.

The late sixties was a time of great confusion for young women. At school, academic teachers prepared us for university and professional careers while the teacher of domestic science, a subject so named to give it more of a scholastic flavour, spent an entire term teaching us to make a wedding cake.

There was also a clash of ideals in the wider world. On one hand, the women's liberation movement was winning hard-fought battles over opportunities for higher education and the chance to pursue a career as a cabinet minister, an academic or a pilot, and on the other, we girls were imbued with centuries of social conditioning that finding Mr Right, breeding, and looking after a house were our preferred destiny. Nobody had yet figured out that it was the freedom to choose any or all of the above options that was the pot of gold.

While my parents were not aficionados of the trap-a-chap scenario, they did want me to be independent and support myself. Consequently, my impassioned bleating at the dinner table about becoming a writer was met with irksome teasing and as much laughter as if I had expressed a desire to become pope. Also, I possessed an unfortunate aptitude for physics and was being steered towards a future of boring atoms by those who knew best.

London Calling

By mid-1970, I was halfway through A levels and I was struggling with too many subjects. One grey, drizzly morning, during Miss Farquhar's pure maths class, I stared out of the window at the rain and it suddenly dawned on me that school was seriously interfering with my education. What I really needed was a Vidal Sassoon haircut, an Ossie Clark dress and a fantastic boyfriend in London.

The major problem I faced, aside from the possible hullabaloo that would come from my parents, was how to effect this change with a healthy swag of O levels, four half-completed A levels, a Raleigh bicycle and the small amount of money I had saved from my Saturday job at a Gosport bakery. In the end, of all things, it was a nosebleed that provided the means of change.

Never before or since has there been such a nosebleed. It was the Trevi Fountain of nosebleeds, and I thought I was going to die. My mother telephoned her friend Jill, who lived next door, and she hurried over. A tall, glamorous woman, Jill assumed an impressive authority, stemmed the flow of my precious bodily fluid, and reassured me with firm but kind words while my mother did the *Times* crossword.

When the drama was over, Jill regaled us with stories of her nursing days at King's College Hospital, and her experiences sounded exciting, fun and very grown-up. And in London, too! The seed was sown, and that night, as I lay in bed, I formulated my plan.

There was, as expected, a great kerfuffle about my decision to abandon school. Reacting as if I were planning to marry a toothless goat herder and live in the Gobi Desert, my mother informed me that I was making a terrible mistake.

'Have you gone completely mad?' she thundered. 'Do you know how many girls would kill to have your education?'

I stared down at the carpet.

'Have you any idea what could happen to you in London?' she went on.

I looked up and nodded. I had, and it all sounded great.

'Don't be smart,' she snapped.

How do they always know what you're thinking?

I couldn't understand why she was so mad. After all, her friend Jill was a state registered nurse, and nursing was a respected profession. Also, if I left home a year earlier than anticipated, Mum could travel the world with my father, who was a master mariner and captain of the *Esso Warwickshire*. Surprised she hadn't thought of this wonderful opportunity, I outlined it for her.

It was the wrong thing to say. My mother became airborne with rage, shouting that university was an opportunity she hadn't had, that student nurses were poorly paid slaves, and that she should have spent more time with me when I was younger.

Mum was playing the guilt card, and I should tell you why.

When I was eight years old and Richard was fourteen, our family suffered the first of two life-changing tragedies. Richard was tobogganing down a snow run on Portsdown Hill when he and the toboggan flew off the slope and landed on a road. Hitting ice, the toboggan careered across the road and slammed into a parked car. Richard's abdomen took the full impact and his insides were badly damaged. Fortunately, Dr Barr-Taylor lived nearby in Leith

Avenue, and he administered life-saving assistance; otherwise, Richard would have died.

My recollections of that time are mostly flashes of traumatic cameos: my rapid delivery to a neighbour's house amid hushed and hurried explanations; my normally bright and laughing mother slumped against a kitchen cupboard, sobbing that Richard was going to die; my father flying home urgently from abroad; Jenny Dog sleeping on Richard's bed and not being shooed off; my grandparents arriving from Liverpool with serious faces; and Mum having a *quiet word* with my teacher at school – memories that terrorized my sleep for a long time.

For Richard, there followed years of hospitalization, agonizing operations and laboured recoveries, and as my father was away at sea for months on end, my brother's care fell on my mother's capable shoulders. She also home-schooled Richard at the kitchen table, determined he was going to recover, finish school and go to university.

To help out, my mother's parents, Leonard and Margaret Higgins, moved from Wallasey near Liverpool to a house close to us in Portchester. Richard and I didn't have paternal grandparents: my father's parents, Joseph and Winifred Johnson, had managed a rubber plantation near Kuala Lumpur in Malaya and had both died before we were born – of what, I have no idea. We knew very little about them, except that our grandfather, Joseph, was once a maths teacher at Malacca High School in what is now Malaysia and was a 'bit of a lad'. Our grandmother, Winifred, was reportedly a real lady and a great friend of the Sultan of Johor, which probably meant she had seen him go past in a car.

My mother's parents were very loving and kind to

me, picking up the parental slack, as Grandpa called it. But they were no match for a lively, inquisitive and imaginative eight-year-old girl who danced to the beat of her own drum – or, as I once heard my mother tell my father, 'It's not just the drum, Herbie J, Maggie's got the whole frigging orchestra in there!' (My father, Herbert Johnson, had been called Herbie J for as long as I'd been alive. My mother, Marion, had been called Brosie since childhood. Clumsy, she would appear with a broken item and announce, 'It's bro!' Over time this morphed into Brosie.)

I must have run my grandparents ragged, but they never complained. Grandpa played a mean game of Monopoly and taught me how to play cribbage, prune roses and wrap apples in newspaper to store for the winter. Nana taught me how to knit, stoke a boiler and make cordial. She baked the best shortbread in Hampshire – in the world, probably.

When my grandfather died of a stroke, then my grandmother of cancer, I was shaken to the core. I was very much left to my own devices after that, and I have to say life was never dull when I was in charge of myself. I viewed many of the sad happenings at home from a safe distance, disappearing into a world of school, books, cycling, swimming and playing tennis with friends each time things got really serious. All I ever recall wanting was for Richard to recover and Mum to buy a television set. It took me ages to wear her down over the television, and then I was only allowed to watch it for an hour a week. While sitting *properly* on a dining-room chair.

Fortunately my mother was a good teacher and my brother an exemplary student, and I'm sure I learned a lot of physics while eavesdropping on Richard's lessons as I prepared dinner under instructions from the kitchen table. I learned to cook, that's for sure, and despite Richard's poor health prognosis he returned to Price's School in Fareham, finished his A levels and secured a place at medical school in Newcastle upon Tyne.

For a long time, Richard was the focus of my mother's existence, but I never felt deprived of attention or doubted that I was loved. Sometimes, though, following the accident, I had felt as if my presence was a nuisance and I was a bit in the way. I had also thought my parents didn't care what I did when I grew up, just as long as I spread my wings and did it somewhere else.

Ha! Turns out I was wrong.

Regardless of my mother's conviction that I was destined for three years of drudgery, servitude and penury, I stood firm on my decision to become a student nurse, and I was happy to report that several of my classmates were planning a similar future. A few girls had mothers who were nursing sisters, and there was a British custom that if your mother had trained at a particular London teaching hospital, then you would follow in her footsteps.

But the tradition didn't end there. At the completion of your training, you would cease work and marry a doctor, produce three children and live in a big house in the country. Somewhere in this grand plan, you would breed Labradors, drive a series of muddy Range Rovers and appear in the spring edition of *Country Life* wearing a twin set and Great Grandma's pearls.

While a few of the class were intent on pursuing

the full catastrophe, I wouldn't be signing up for any of the post-training malarkey. Come to think of it, I wouldn't be following in my mother's footsteps either. Of all things, my extraordinary mother was an armoured tank mechanic in the Wrens.

Disbanded in 1919, the Wrens were revived in 1939 at the beginning of the Second World War, and my mother had joined up. Her career as a mechanic was obviously motivated and defined by that dreadful war, and I imagine she saw too much horror during those years because, like my father, she was reluctant to speak about it. In a box in the attic, there were black-and-white photographs of her in military uniform smiling that 'everything is going splendidly' expression they all trumped up for the cameras, but that is all.

In fact, the only obvious legacy of my mother's career was her ability to repair armoured tanks and lawnmowers. Wisely, I refrained from pointing out that nursing would bestow broader skills on me.

An apparent disappointment to my family, my teachers and our daily cleaner, I was left alone to contact the School of Nursing at King's College Hospital, fill in the forms, arrange referees, and pay for suitable clothing and the train fare to London if there was an interview.

'No way is Maggie going to be a nurse,' Richard told anyone who would listen. 'She hasn't completed her A levels, so King's won't consider her.'

Essentially, this was true. Gaining entry to a school of nursing at a London teaching hospital was highly competitive, and the intake favoured girls with three A levels. But nothing ventured, nothing gained, and the sibling vote of no confidence made me more determined than ever to be a nurse.

There is no doubt in my mind that the harmless lie I promoted in my application to the prestigious School of Nursing at King's wasn't nearly as underhand as the surprise ward allocation they were lining up for me.

What was my harmless lie?

Well, it's quite simple. I fibbed in the covering letter that I was descended from a long line of dedicated nurses and had dreamed of being a nurse since I was three years old. For good measure, I mentioned there was a distinct possibility that mine was a spiritual calling.

Too much?

Not at all. A week later, a letter arrived from King's advising that the intake was full, but late applicants would be interviewed and considered if a vacancy became available. A date and time for me to attend was noted.

Now they would see for themselves the makings of a terrific nurse. My imagination went into overdrive. In the first year of training, I would save the life of somebody important and Matron's admiration would be immeasurable. Truly, the possibilities for glory were endless.

No one was prouder than me when the day of the interview arrived. Keen as mustard, and with the supreme confidence of youth, I took the train from Fareham to Waterloo station. Outside, I hopped on a red double-decker bus to King's at Denmark Hill. It was high summer and devilishly warm, and I felt very sophisticated and worldly as I sat upstairs amid thick cigarette smoke and admired my reflection in the grubby bus window.

My teenage reverie was short-lived. No sooner had

I stepped off the bus at the hospital than the supreme confidence of youth took a nosedive down the nearest drain. I had been expecting a lovely old gabled building at the end of a sweeping drive lined with flowering roses, and maybe a pretty nurse wearing a cape and a white veil pushing an injured soldier in a wheelchair across a lawn. The picture in front of me wasn't right at all. Across the busy road stood a massive, imposing brick and stone edifice. It was the largest hospital I had ever seen, like Buckingham Palace for ill people. And there wasn't a rose in sight.

Suddenly a nurse dashed past me. She sprinted over the road, through the black wrought-iron gates, and across the hospital forecourt before mounting steps and disappearing through a side door. Following in hot pursuit, I found myself in a lounge area packed with nurses just a little older than me. They were chatting and laughing and drinking from white cups. I thought they looked smashing in their uniforms – mature, attractive and self-assured. One girl was smoking a black cigarette with a gold tip. Another had kicked off her shoes and was sitting sideways in the chair with her legs dangling over the arm. What sophistication! What class! I *so* wanted to be a part of that scene.

Shaking like a whippet, I sat on a hard wooden chair in an enormous sitting room under the highest ceiling in the world and faced two of the most frightening old women I had ever seen. Starch-stiff and baggy-bosomed, they were wearing dark-green nurse uniforms with white cuffs and collars. Each wore a white linen bonnet perched atop her tightly permed head. I could smell lavender eau-de-Cologne. They could probably smell fear.

After staring at me for some time, the Zeppelin-sized one on the right, whom I guessed was the top banana, demanded, 'Why do you want to be a nurse, Miss Johnson?' Her voice would have frozen spinach.

I swallowed hard and looked straight at her. Fortune favours those who have prepared and, ever the Girl Guide (leader of Fuchsia Patrol), I was ready for this question. 'I've always wanted to be a nurse and care for the sick,' I lied boldly. 'I think it's the most brilliant thing.' Then I sighed and glanced coyly down as though imparting a secret. 'For as long as I can remember, it's all I've ever wanted to do.'

Miraculously, lightning didn't strike me dead.

Both women continued to stare, and I was convinced they had seen through my act. At seventeen, I was unsure of the world and the people in it, and I worried the hospital might have some sort of secret government access to my teachers and personal diaries. My entire knowledge of technology was informed by *Dr Who*, so to me anything was possible.

Anticipating a grilling, I squirmed on the chair, fiddled with the hem of my purpose-bought Marks & Spencer skirt, and hoped an unexploded bomb would be found in the car park and we'd all have to be evacuated.

'Nursing is a vocation,' the top banana abruptly announced. 'It is held in high regard and requires strength of character, commitment to hard work and adherence to the values of the profession. It is not for the faint-hearted!'

Far out. This was amazing. I was exactly what they were looking for.

But then came the question I was dreading.

'Why don't you wait another year and finish your A levels?'

Hmm? Uneasy ground. Explaining that I was desperate to pursue my calling, I asked if they would take into consideration my current academic achievements. For icing, I threw in the Human Biology AO level (a syllabus graded between O and A levels) that I had recently acquired and my Royal Society of the Arts Mathematics award, which a garden gnome could have passed. It sounded impressive, but it wasn't three completed A levels.

There was more scribbling and then the bottom banana asked if I was in good health. I replied that I was, and she asked if I was married or engaged. Honestly, I plumb near fell off the chair at that one. Picturing my mother helpless with laughter, I couldn't hide a grin.

Mistaking my expression for cheek, the top banana looked disapproving and explained with almost evangelical fervour that only single women who were committed to the rigours of the *exceptional clinical nurse training offered at King's College Hospital* would be considered. This was accompanied by a sterling dissertation on the privilege bestowed on those girls allowed to grace the hallowed floors of King's world-renowned wards.

Suitably chastised, I pretended to look thoughtful while my future lay in their chapped, ringless hands. Eventually the top banana leaned forward and told me that a girl had recently withdrawn her application, and as I would soon turn eighteen, and there was now an unexpected vacancy in the September set, I could start in a few weeks.

I tried not to appear exuberant while the bottom

banana explained that I would live in the nurses' home, be provided with uniforms and laundering of same, receive an allowance, and spend the first eight weeks in PTS at the School of Nursing, where I would learn anatomy, physiology and basic nursing procedures. She didn't mention that it would be some time before I actually set foot on one of those celebrated wards at King's College Hospital.

'You can go,' the top banana said dismissively.

I stood up. 'Thank you,' I said, and smiled triumphantly.

A short time after the interview, I changed into brown suede hot pants, a lime-green polyester top and plat-form shoes. To complete the transformation, I applied lashings of blue mascara and pale pink lipstick.

Looking like an accident in a paint factory, I caught a bus to Marble Arch, purchased a lava lamp in Selfridges and, with a renewed sense of purpose, pranced up and down Oxford Street like I owned the place.

Later, I learned that the tutors at King's School of Nursing were attending a meeting elsewhere, and as I was the only latecomer to be interviewed, the task had been handed to any available ward sisters.

I was too young to know that my silly lie in the application letter didn't matter. And I would come to learn that the important consideration was that I was healthy and strong and, at hardly any cost, could be allocated to work in areas of the hospital that were difficult to staff. I also looked like the sort of girl who would do as she was told.

To this end, I had surprise on my side . . .

*

It was early evening when I caught the train home. My face hurt from smiling and I was bone-tired. Leaning a cheek against the window, I watched the familiar green hills of the South Downs roll past.

Before reaching Fareham, I removed the make-up, changed back into the interview clothes and tidied my hair. Our house was a half-hour walk from the station, and I couldn't wait to get home, sit sideways on a chair and dangle my legs elegantly over the arm.

As I approached our house, I could see my mother tinkering with the lawnmower on the driveway. Our pooch, Jenny Dog, was standing at the front gate with her head poking through the metal uprights. A light mist from the hose was drifting across the lawn, and a thrush was perched on the garden fork to which the hose was tied: the usual reassuring rhythms of home.

Seeing me, Mum stood up and pressed her hand into the small of her back, as she always did, to counteract the bend. Smiling, she asked, 'Well, did you tell them to get lost?'

'Err . . . not exactly,' I mumbled.

Then all hell broke loose.

'You'll be a slave,' she shouted furiously. 'A char!' Incandescent with rage, she wrung her hands in frustration. 'I should never have let you attend the interview! I thought it would put you off! Oh, sweet Jesus!'

In short succession, my mother had me stabbed in a dark alley, on drugs and pregnant with twins. Angrily, she kicked the lawnmower. The thrush hastily abandoned the garden fork and Jenny Dog suddenly had pressing canine business in the back garden. Great. I was alone with Cruella de Vil.

There was no point arguing about my decision. It was best to go inside, make a pot of tea, sit down and calmly discuss my plans. Yes, that was the mature way to handle this. So I ran to my bedroom and slammed the door. No supper. No *Z Cars*. My life in ruins.

Where were my brother and father while this drama unfolded?

Thankfully, my brother was hundreds of miles away working as a houseman (junior doctor) at the Royal Victoria Infirmary in Newcastle, and my father was safely manoeuvring his oil tanker somewhere off the coast of Valparaíso, Chile. But unfortunately the home guard was on the premises, and a short time later my mother entered my room and sat on the bed beside me. Pulling me towards her, she kissed the side of my face.

'You're such a gladiator,' she said. 'I just want you to understand that you will be a general dogsbody for at least a year.'

I cast my eyes upwards. What did she know?

Quite a lot, as it turned out. And who among us was ever going to report that satisfying confirmation back to base?

Certainly not me.

CHAPTER 3

What the Dickens?

Preliminary Training School, London: Autumn 1970

IT WAS 2 A.M. on a wet and windy morning, and a fuzzy-edged moon shone hazily down on Hambledon House, the rambling old mansion of a nurses' home in South London where many new King's student nurses, including me, were locked up at night.

Situated in the well-to-do suburb of Dulwich Village, the home was surrounded by Dulwich Golf Course, Dulwich Park and Dulwich College, and had been bequeathed to King's by W. H. Smith, the bookshop people. The secluded location deemed the property a perfect billet for virginal young girls entrusted to the hospital's care. No one owned a car, there was no public transport in the village, and the home was far from pubs, discos and men. There was absolutely no possibility of shenanigans.

Or so they thought . . .

'I *love* you, Miranda,' wailed a drunken male voice in the front garden. 'I looove you . . .'

'Ssssh!' Miranda hissed at Danny, from a first-floor window. 'You'll wake the warden!'

'But I looove you,' Danny swooned back. 'I really,

really love you . . . and I'm all wet . . . and the door's locked.'

'Oh, for goodness' sake,' Miranda said crossly. 'Who shut the front door?'

Who indeed?

We were not provided with keys to the front door, an entry point overseen by a female warden whose job it was to keep us safe. Habitually, after she had locked up at night and downed a stiff cocoa, a student nurse would tiptoe to the front door and wedge it ajar with a black nursing shoe. There were no security alarms or closed-circuit cameras, and the shoe allowed us and our guests the freedom to come and go at night.

If the warden were to discover our clever ruse, she would have a hard time figuring out who owned the shoe. We had all been sledgehammered into purchasing two pairs of identical black leather nursing shoes, called K-Skips, which no doubt provided a healthy backhander for someone but also gave each shoe's owner complete anonymity. The only downside to our scheme was that you didn't always get your shoe back.

'Hey, Miranda! Let me in!' Danny demanded. Then he belched loudly.

A slender green-eyed girl with long wavy fair hair, Miranda had been dating Danny for ages – almost three weeks. She made it to the vestibule quick smart, having thrown on her dressing-gown and K-Skips, and opened the front door.

But she was too late. The warden, looking very East End in a pink candlewick dressing-gown and a chiffon scarf over her curlers, was right behind her, and she was holding a black nursing shoe.

'I found this shoe propping the door open earlier,' the warden said angrily. 'Is it yours?'

Miranda pointed down at her shoes. 'No, I'm wearing mine.'

Seeing his girlfriend, Danny staggered forwards. 'Oh, Miranda, there you are,' he sang happily. 'Is this your mother?'

Looking at Miranda, the warden pointed at Danny. 'Well, then, is he yours?'

'I've never seen him before in my life,' Miranda responded curtly, and walked swiftly away.

'Oh dear.' Danny wailed. Then he tripped backwards and fell into a rhododendron bush.

Shortly, the front door closed and the only sounds were of distant thunder and rain splattering the driveway. I know this because I was behind the rhododendron bush with my boyfriend, Kip. Also unable to enter the nurses' home, and soaked to the skin, we were huddled under Kip's second-hand army greatcoat, helpless with laughter.

Danny and Kip were university students at King's College London, Danny studying law and Kip medicine. Danny's girlfriend, Miranda, who was a nurse in my set and with whom I had already become friends, had stayed at home to study for a test while the rest of us had gone partying at the hospital rugby club a couple of miles away on Dog Kennel Hill. Known as 'Doggers', the knockabout clubhouse served cheap drinks, played good dance music and had fast become our regular haunt. High on beer and youthful exuberance, Kip, Danny and I were three sheets to the wind, and Danny just had to see Miranda.

But what to do? The only phone was on the other

side of the front door, and we had spent our last cash on chips and pickled onions. There was nothing left for a cab, and credit cards were a pipe-dream away. Meanwhile, the rain was becoming heavier.

'I'm gonna break a window,' Danny announced, and struggled to stand. Kip and I helped him up and then we all fell down.

'I could walk him back to hall,' Kip suggested. They both lived at the King's hall of residence on Champion Hill, a fair hike away.

'And I'll just lie here in the garden, shall I, looking like a crime scene?' I said, and we burst out laughing again.

'Sssh!' Kip hissed, but no one could have heard us over the rain. Lying there, I hoped Miranda would sneak back down and unlock the door, but she didn't. Later, she told me she hadn't dared.

But salvation was at hand. A young man holding an umbrella was running up the driveway. I recognized him immediately. It was Fraser, my friend Adele's husband, who was illegally living with Adele in her room at Hambledon House. Keeping their marriage secret and hiding Fraser was the only way they could negotiate the rules that married women couldn't train to be nurses, and that new student nurses *must* live in the nurses' home. Adele was determined to be a nurse, and I envied and admired her courage in challenging the archaic system.

Fraser informed us that Adele had left a window open round the back, and that he would run Kip and Danny home in his car, which he'd parked up the road. Relieved, I watched Kip and Fraser struggle down the driveway with a rubber-legged Danny between them.

Drenched to the bone and shivering so much my teeth were chattering, I nipped round the back and climbed in through the window. Once in my room, I dried off, crept down to the hall and wedged the front door open for other latecomers.

Almost immediately, another girl from my set, Polly, came charging in. A comely lass with a mop of light-brown curls framing her serene and gentle face, Polly had been to a party in Herne Hill with her medical-student boyfriend, James.

'Thanks, Maggie!' Polly said cheerfully, and gave me a peck on the cheek before disappearing off to her room.

It goes without saying that a small group of us frequently had hangovers during those early weeks of our training, and sometimes no sleep at all. And I only had three shoes at the end of PTS.

Hard to believe, I know.

As soon as I could, I apologized to the other Nurse Johnson for sneaking away from class. Gracious in the extreme, she chuckled and informed me that she had no idea what it was about as our tutor had soon realized the mistake. And the story gets better. Unbelievably, her first name was also Margaret. Oh, what fortune could be mine from having the same name as another nurse?

In this case, quite a lot. The other Margaret Johnson was a delightful, dark-haired girl with the kindest eyes, the warmest smile, and the softest, honeyed voice in the world. She was the type of girl who made grown men want to catch something serious just so they could be looked after by her. I could already hear my name being given high praise in professional circles.

Margaret and I agreed to address potential

confusion in a simple way. Her middle name was Frances and mine was Judith, and as there was already a Judith in our set, to our friends and colleagues she would be 'Fran' and I would be 'Maggie' – although I have an idea she was always a Fran because it suited her.

Even more unbelievably, I wasn't reprimanded over any of my misdemeanours, and the issue over the dog wasn't mentioned again – at least, not *that* dog disaster. There was, I cannot lie, an even better one brewing . . .

In 1970, student-nurse training in Britain was hospital-based and overseen by a senior nurse tutor, a position later titled director of nurse education. In our case, the DNE was a sweet-faced woman called Sister Caroline, who spoke with a hint of a German accent.

Ward sisters at King's College Hospital (referred to as King's or KCH) were known by a Christian name that wasn't always their own, and we were lucky pups to have Sister Caroline watching over us. A velvet rock, she was kind and thoughtful towards students: two characteristics that set her apart from many ward sisters, who felt we were better served by public humiliation delivered with a Gatling gun.

Quaintly referred to as Nightingale Training, the accepted theory behind the hospital-based model was that student nurses gained knowledge and practical experience while working on the wards. Ostensibly supervised by a ward sister or tutor, students were included as part of the staffing allocation (not supernumerary, as I believe we should have been) and rotated through different disciplines such as medical, surgical, theatre, casualty, orthopaedics and so on. To complete our education, the ward work was supported by periodic blocks of theoretical and practical instruction held at the School of Nursing.

PTS kept regular hours, and Monday to Friday we dressed in our uniforms, packed *Toohey's Medicine for Nurses* in our bags and were bussed to the School of Nursing at Dulwich Hospital, a short distance away.

Dulwich Hospital?

'We should be at King's,' a student in the front seat told the bus driver on our first day.

'Not any more,' he said, amused by our confusion. 'Dulwich, St Giles and St Francis merged with King's four years ago to become King's College Hospital Group. The nursing schools have merged too, so you all have to get off. Come along. Chop-chop!'

There was a collective murmur of dissent.

'I'm sure this isn't right!' Jan complained.

'I refuse to get off!' Adele stated firmly.

'I'm going to telephone my father,' an upper-crust voice announced. 'He's a consultant at St Thomas' Hospital.'

'Ooooooooooh!' mocked the rest of us.

Our threats fell on deaf ears, and eventually we got off the bus and traipsed into Dulwich Hospital.

In class, with the aid of a plastic skeleton and charts, tutors shared with us the joys of anatomy and physiology. We practised giving bed-baths and bedpans while guarding our patients' privacy, and we learned to make beds efficiently. We charted patient observations, checking temperatures with a mercury thermometer and counting pulse beats and respirations per minute against the second hands on our shiny new fob watches.

We monitored blood pressure with a sphygmoma-nometer (a machine that took longer to learn how to spell than to use) and were taught that normal blood pressure was a hundred plus your age over eighty. (Today, normal blood pressure is rated lower – a cynic might think a market needed to be found for new blood-pressure medications.)

We operated suction machines, oxygen cylinders and autoclaves, changed IV bottles and bags, bandaged limbs and digits, tepid-sponged imaginary fevers, gained knowledge on bedsore prevention and treatments, discovered the intricacies of barrier-nursing the infectious, prepared inhalations, memorized indwelling catheter care and mouth care, and practised methods of lifting patients.

Once a week, we received a lecture from a doctor, which was our nap time, and we were shown short films on instrument sterilization, venereal disease (not good before lunch), the kiss of life (CPR), last offices (laying out a dead body), injections, wound care and nutrition.

At Dulwich Hospital, we practised ward evacuation and how to operate fire extinguishers (very satisfying), were taken on visits to the modern wards and operating theatres at King's (very impressive), toured the mortuary (very sobering) and sat stiff with horror as an esteemed surgeon advised that one in ten of us would die of breast cancer.

Board and lodging was deducted from our meagre monthly allowance. Lunch at Dulwich Hospital was decent, but breakfast and dinner at Hambledon House were abysmal, with only two choices: take it or leave it. To avoid starvation, the Chinese nurses bought ingredients and a camping stove and cooked sensational-smelling meals in their rooms. For a while, there was mean-spirited talk of ducks disappearing in Dulwich Park, but I never believed the rumour, especially as I had started it.

On the health front, tuberculosis (TB) was a common infectious disease in Britain, so we had chest X-rays and received a range of vaccinations. In class, we took written, oral and practical tests, and attended our half-day shifts on the wards, where, under the supposed supervision of the ward sister, we were building on information and practical applications learned in class. Except on Dickens I wasn't building anything except muscles. Apart from one partial bed-bath and the disastrous tea round, all I did was clean.

What were the real cleaners doing? Stuff all, as far as I could see. In between hanging out of the bathroom window smoking and dusting invisible cobwebs from the ceiling, they dawdled around behind a cleaning machine the size of a small hovercraft and polished the same spot over and over again in front of the television in the day room.

Our weekends were earmarked for serious study, and my friends and I threw off our paper caps and went to the pub. We tried on dresses that we couldn't afford in Harrods, hung around under Marble Arch and pretended to be foreigners asking for directions, jeered the lunatics at Speakers' Corner, walked and ran and laughed in Kew Gardens, and searched for bargains in Carnaby Street.

Of the fifty-eight students in my set, all were young and female, and many hailed from markedly different backgrounds to my safe, middle-class upbringing. Until London, I had lived among people like me, played sports with people like me and, apart

What the Dickens?

from my Saturday job at a Gosport bakery, mixed and studied with people like me. Suddenly I was in a melting pot: Chinese, Canadians, Indians, West Indians, Scots, Irish, Welsh and English.

Poorly paid, far from home, and without the benefit of an active student union, we had to support each other. The shared adversity of poverty bred in us a strong sense of loyalty, and within a few weeks we had established firm friendships, many forged at Hambledon House, where I was lucky to share an attic room with Kathy and Laurel.

I was drawn to Kathy's warm-hearted personality from the start. A gentle, loose-limbed girl with masses of wavy brown hair, she had a captivating Brummie accent and everyone was attracted to her sweet vulnerability. Having left her large family and boyfriend, Dave, in Birmingham, Kathy had come to London to spread her wings. Creatively inclined, she talked with longing of the bright hippy lights of San Francisco.

Laurel had the bed next to mine, and we grew on each other slowly. A buxom, fair-haired Canadian girl, she came across as larger than life, but behind the out-there façade she was shy to the point of climbing into bed to change into her pyjamas. Short-sighted, she wore thick spectacles that made her eyes look like golf balls, and, rather startlingly, they were often the first thing I saw every morning when she shook me awake. A natural comedian, she could have us all in fits of laughter in a trice. Like Kathy, Laurel had a boyfriend back home, except her man was in Canada. She missed him dreadfully and there were frequently tears at night.

In the attic room next to ours was another Canadian, Meredith. A striking girl with straight black hair styled in a bob, she had brown, almond-shaped eyes and smooth white skin, and was, I think, more career-orientated than the rest of us. There was a resolute neatness about her that I admired, and I think she secretly envied my bohemian ways as we became good friends.

St Giles Hospital was grim.

Years of preservation and renewal had turned the sturdy old red-brick buildings with their white-edged windows into an architectural hotchpotch of admin offices, ward blocks of varying levels, a nurses' home and a strange five-storey tower of circular wards – all the rage at the time, apparently.

Dickens was an older ward and could have done with a visit from Laura Ashley. Iron-frame beds were spaced evenly around the yellowing walls, and between each bed was a dismal privacy curtain, a large bare window, a metal locker and a brown *faux*-leather armchair. At the ward entrance were the kitchen, linen room, sister's office and clinical room, and at the far end a communal bathroom and sluice. There were no showers, and patients had a regular bath or bed-bath, or were given a bowl of hot water if they were able to wash themselves but couldn't get out of bed.

I had one more half-day on Dickens before I was to take my final PTS exam, which I was sure to fail unless there were questions on cleaning products. And I wasn't even having supervision with that. What if I mixed together two chemicals that exploded and burned down the hospital? I mean, I had certainly thought about it.

Apprehensive as I walked on to the ward, I was relieved to see Rosie O'Brien on duty. I had no notion that this morning, instead of cleaning, I was to practise real nursing care and learn something that would define the ethos of King's.

Nobody knew the age of One-Ear Jones. Not even One-Ear Jones. Somewhere around seventy, he lived under the overhang of a lockup in an alleyway behind an Indian restaurant in Peckham Rye. Brought in by ambulance, Mr Jones had been on a bender for five days and was found in the alleyway soaking wet and barely conscious. Dr Freeman, the houseman who admitted Mr Jones to Dickens, had written 'hypothermia' as the diagnosis. TLC was the treatment noted, which meant a hot bath, delousing, clean clothes, hot food and a warm bed, all provided with tender loving care.

I didn't realize it, but I was being shown the true benevolence, brilliance and humanity of the National Health Service. Started in Britain in 1948, four years before I was born, the NHS provided free top-of-the-range health care to everyone in the country, regardless of wealth. I had no idea this wasn't the case in other Western countries.

Sister Morag was attending a meeting, so Rosie asked me to help her bath Mr Jones. Pleased, I pushed the wheelchair carrying him into the bathroom, and I have to tell you he smelt eye-wateringly horrendous. From her pocket, Rosie produced a bottle of Yardley English Lavender and dabbed some under her nose. She offered me the fragrance, which I gladly applied.

'What's that?' Mr Jones asked Rosie.

'Scent,' she told him.

He grabbed the bottle from me, took a healthy swig and wiped his mouth with the back of his hand.

'Hey!' Rosie cried out. 'That costs money, you know!'

'Sorry, Nurse,' Mr Jones said, not looking at all sorry.

'Won't that make him sick?' I asked Rosie, concerned.

She shook her head. 'I doubt it. I'm sure Mr Jones will tell us if he feels poorly.'

Lord save us, I could see bugs hopping about on his head. I had no idea how I was going to touch him – there was a possibility of disease on every part of his being.

Rosie, on the other hand, didn't appear concerned. Humming away, she put the plug in the bath, tipped in a handful of Lux flakes to help soak off the scabs and dirt, ran the taps, and tested the temperature with her hand until the bath was three-quarters full of hot, soapy water.

Big enough to hold a pregnant rhinoceros, the above-floor bath was in the middle of the room, allowing patients to be tended by a nurse on each side. Rosie closed the high windows to keep Mr Jones warm, and they quickly steamed up.

'Now, Mr Jones,' Rosie said, 'we have sick patients on Dickens, and Nurse Johnson and I are going to cover ourselves so you don't pick up germs.'

'If you say so,' he mumbled.

Rosie beckoned me outside, where we replaced our headwear with paper theatre hats to protect our hair, and both put on surgical gloves and white gowns over our uniforms.

'Apart from being a drunk, what's the matter with him?' I asked Rosie, as we secured the ties behind each other's gowns.

'Oh, don't say that,' she chided. 'He's just a homeless old man who needs looking after.'

'But he's taking up the bed of someone who is genuinely ill,' I said with certainty. 'It's his own fault he's like he is.'

Rosie looked horrified. 'He's a human being,

Maggie,' she thundered angriliy, 'and it's not for you to make judgements on him or his care. Every person who comes through the door of this hospital deserves respect, no matter who they are, the state they are in, or where they have come from.'

My righteous indignation silenced, I was embarrassed and a little annoyed by Rosie's sudden hostility. Surely it *was* One-Ear Jones's own fault that he was in the state he was in?

'And while we're at it,' Rosie went on, still angry, 'Mr Jones has probably already swallowed a bottle of methylated spirits this morning, so a bit of lavender water won't hurt him.'

'Oh,' was all I could manage in response.

Methylated spirits, Yardley English Lavender, Lux flakes . . . No one was going to believe this.

Sheepishly, I followed Rosie back into the bathroom, determined to recover friendly ground.

'Hello again, sir,' I said to Mr Jones. 'You're going to feel like a new man after a nice hot bath.'

'Don't overdo it,' Rosie whispered, and when I saw her grin I smiled back.

'I'll keep my undies on, if you don't mind,' Mr Jones said, as we helped him undress.

As I peeled off Mr Jones's socks, some skin came away from his heels. I retched and Rosie said matter-of-factly, 'That happens sometimes, Maggie. Just get on with it.'

Pulling myself together, I helped Rosie lift Mr Jones into the bath. As we stood him up, he released a blast of wind at alarming velocity.

'Never mind, Mr Jones,' Rosie said cheerfully. 'That could happen to anyone.'

Keeping our heads as far from his as we could, we

lowered him into the bath. Water sloshed like Niagara over the sides on to our shoes.

Mr Jones was a mess. In addition to scabies, he was covered with weeping sores, scabs and caked-on who-knows-what. His hair was matted, and his beard was long and full of dirt. His finger- and toenails were so long they had curled over. And his underpants were so soiled and threadbare that they fell apart in the water.

'If it's all right with you, Mr Jones,' Rosie said, 'we will give you clean clothes and wash your others so they'll be clean for tomorrow.'

He nodded. 'Put them where I can see them,' he said. 'I don't want anyone stealing my things.'

Rosie lifted the clothes off the floor and placed them in a plastic bag before putting it where Mr Jones could see it. We trimmed his hair and beard with surgical scissors and gently washed him from top to toe, using a jug to rinse his hair. After carefully cutting his finger- and toenails, we drained the bath, refilled it with hot water, added handfuls of salt, and then washed him all over again with Fairy soap. Discreetly, Rosie lifted out bits of underpants that had come away. I couldn't bring myself to touch them.

'I'm sure Mr Jones would rather have Klaus dry and dress him than us,' Rosie said, and she winked at me.

Immediately, I understood why. If Mr Jones hadn't wanted to take his undies off in front of us, then there was no way he would let us wash his bottom and between his legs. This was a great relief.

Klaus was a German conscientious objector, known as a 'conchie'. Tall and lanky, with a super-hero square jaw and a deep, guttural voice, he was unwilling to serve the German military in any capacity and, with the approval of his government, he had chosen instead to work as an orderly in a foreign hospital. Luckily, he had chosen ours.

'You'll like Klaus,' Rosie told Mr Jones. 'He's Dutch.'

'No, he's not, Rosie,' I said, without thinking. 'He's German.'

'I'm not having a Jerry touch me,' Mr Jones complained. Mortified, I realized why Rosie had said Klaus was Dutch. Oh, what an idiot.

'Klaus is a conscientious objector,' Rosie explained. 'A pacifist.'

Mr Jones looked thoughtful, I think tossing up which was worse: a German conchie touching him or two girls seeing his privates.

'Does he smoke? I like a man who smokes,' Mr Jones asked.

'Like a chimney,' Rosie assured him. I knew Klaus didn't smoke. I was learning from Rosie, even though a few of her ideas were, I felt, misguided.

'Then I'll allow Klaus to help me,' Mr Jones decided, and Rosie went to find him.

Shortly, she returned with Klaus.

'*Guten Morgen, Herr Jones,*' Klaus said, in his thick German accent, and Mr Jones rudely ignored him. Klaus leaned forward and felt Mr Jones's pulse. Then he felt his own pulse and said in alarm, 'Oh, *mein Gott im Himmel*. It is me, ze Kraut, who is dead!'

One-Ear Jones looked up at Klaus and a smile spread across his weather-beaten old face. 'You'll do,' he said.

After giving Klaus instructions on covering Mr Jones with benzyl benzoate to treat the scabies before dressing him, Rosie slipped her cigarettes and lighter into Klaus's pocket. 'Let him have one in the bath,' she whispered, as we left the bathroom.

At the nurses' desk, the admitting houseman, Dr Freeman, was looking for One-Ear Jones.

'How is he?' he wanted to know.

'Cleaner,' Rosie said.

Nodding approval, Freeman leaned against the desk. A big man with curly brown hair, he reminded me of the actor Elliott Gould. 'Do you nurses know his history?' he asked.

We shook our heads.

'He was a GP in London before the war,' Freeman explained. 'His house and surgery were bombed during the Blitz, and he lost his mother, wife and their three children.'

Shocked, I asked, 'Is that how he lost his ear? In the Blitz?'

'No,' Dr Freeman said. 'He lit a cigarette while drinking methylated spirits and the explosion sent his ear halfway across Lewisham.'

'Oh, my goodness!' I gasped.

Out of the corner of my eye, I saw Sister Morag bearing down on us. Clapping her hands at us as if we were children, she scolded, 'Enough chatting! And I'll thank you not to lean on the furniture, Dr Freeman.'

'I tried to lean on the nurses,' he teased her, 'but they wouldn't let me.' Ignoring the fire in Sister Morag's eyes, he thanked Rosie and me – we were grinning like Cheshire cats – and sauntered off.

'We were discussing a patient,' Rosie told Sister Morag, with daring resentment.

'Back to work,' Sister Morag growled. 'And wipe those stupid smiles off your faces!'

What the Dickens?

As we scrubbed the bath, I apologized to Rosie for thinking that Mr Jones was taking up the bed of someone who genuinely needed it.

'Oh dear, you still don't get it, do you?' She sighed. 'Now you think that because he was a doctor and lost his family it's okay for him to have a bed.'

'Well, yes,' I said, dismayed.

Rosie shook her head. 'It wouldn't matter if he was a thief or a prince. Everyone who walks through the hospital doors receives the same respectful treatment. It's what underpins King's, Maggie. It's what's right.'

By the end of PTS, I hadn't practised much nursing on the ward, but I had learned a valuable lesson in humanity. Worried about passing the PTS exam, I studied my lecture notes until I had done all I could. If I failed, so be it. I had made some great friends, I had a Vidal Sassoon haircut, an Ossie Clark dress and a London boyfriend, Kip, the King's medical student. Kip was tall, dark-haired and knee-tremblingly dishy. It remained to be seen if he was fantastic or not, as per my master plan.

We had a week off before finding out if we had passed our PTS exam and could start full-time training. As my parents were in Cape Town, I hitched home to Fareham with Laurel and Miranda. We walked across the water-meadows in the wind and rain, played Fleetwood Mac, Bob Dylan and Joni Mitchell records at full volume, and drank Guinness by the open fire. When the Guinness ran out, we caught the train to Miranda's home in Marlow and walked beside the Thames. We were talking and laughing so much we could have been walking on Mars.

Somehow, while revelling in the waning light of

the peace, love and flower-power movement of the sixties, and celebrating the freedom of our new lives in the dawn of seventies London, my friends and I had passed our PTS nursing exams.

Jan, Laurel, Miranda, Polly, Tilly, Adele, Kathy and Meredith couldn't wait to start full-time on their wards.

Me?

I dreaded returning to Dickens and dreamed of nursing at King's on wards such as Pantia Ralli, Annie Zunz, Trundle and Waddington, Twining . . . oh, the wonderful names.

Quite frankly, something had to be done.

CHAPTER 4

Just Get On with It

St Giles Hospital, London: November 1970

I STARTED WORK as a full-time first-year student nurse on Dickens with a heavy heart and a wee bit of a hangover.

Clutching at straws, I had asked at the School of Nursing if I could be moved to another ward and was told to report to Dickens or leave. I chose the former, telling myself I was a child of post-war, ration-ridden England and had endured worse hardships. There was Viking blood in my veins, for goodness' sake. I could do this.

Or was I staying to save face? Or hanging on because I had made good friends, had a boyfriend and loved London? Who knows? One thing was certain, though: if Dickens was real nursing, I hated it.

As a reward to myself for staying, I bought my first maxi skirt in Petticoat Lane, and to deter self-indulgent pity I started reading *The Female Eunuch* by Germaine Greer. I was enjoying the book, but it probably wasn't the best reading material for a girl embarking on a profession that specialized in the suppression of women.

There had been a few changes on Dickens. Two patients had transferred to St Francis and four men had died. Unfortunately, each had been replaced with an identical old man. But, miracle of miracles, two patients had gone home! Mr Gribble, the fox-hunting man, had been discharged with medicine to treat his thyroid condition, and One-Ear Jones had been packed off to his alleyway in Peckham Rye with an old sleeping bag of Dr Freeman's and a packet of Rosie's cigarettes. Amazingly, apart from liver damage due to his habit of constantly irrigating himself with alcohol, which the hospital couldn't resolve without his compliance, there was nothing seriously wrong with him.

I was distressed to find that my favourite patient, Mr Clegg, was extremely frail. Rosie explained that his heart muscle was weaker and could no longer pump blood efficiently around his body. He was retaining fluid and his lungs were congested, and on top of his congestive cardiac failure an X-ray had revealed a tumour on his right lung. Owing to his fragile health and advanced age (ninety-three), active treatment for the tumour, such as surgery or intensive radiation, had been considered unkind and not in Mr Clegg's best interests.

In the next bed to Mr Clegg's, the oh-so-odious Mr Snape was still in residence. With good nursing care, antibiotics and chest physiotherapy, he had recovered from influenza and bronchitis, but he'd suffered a small stroke before he could be transferred to St Francis. He was recovering from the stroke and, according to Rosie, was now more of a bad-tempered mouse than a ferocious lion.

It was fairly routine in 1970 for elderly male patients to be tested for syphilis, which they might have contracted during the Second World War. Left untreated, as many cases were, syphilis had the potential to develop into what was known as general paralysis of the insane (GPI), a neurological disorder that caused muscular deterioration and symptoms of dementia. None of our men had GPI, but it's likely that some had undiagnosed dementia or post-traumatic stress disorder (PTSD), particularly those who awoke screaming from a snooze. Personally, I think it was relevant that many of them were selective in whom they abused, their targets being exclusively young women. Hence my diagnosis: acute misogynous stinkerism (AMS).

Rosie O'Brien and Ursula Tibbs (a third-year student nurse) handled the abuse with an entertaining double act that cheered me up as I was wiping down Mr Barlow's bedside locker.

'How are you today, Mr Barlow?' Rosie gaily called to him, as she sailed past with a vomit bowl.

'Mind your own effing business!' Mr Barlow shouted back.

Two seconds later, Ursula passed us carrying blankets and called, 'Just minding my own effing business, Mr Barlow.'

'Bleedin' Abbott and Costello,' he yelled at Ursula's back.

Eighty-year-old Mr Barlow had rheumatoid arthritis and was admitted for three weeks' respite care while his wife, who looked after him at home, had her gall bladder removed at Dulwich Hospital.

'I wouldn't be surprised,' Ursula confided to Rosie and me in the sluice, 'if Mrs Barlow arranged to have something removed every few months just to get away from her husband.'

'At least until she runs out of spare parts,' Rosie quipped.

Another new admission, Wilfred Hyde, was an angry eighty-four-year-old with hypertension, diabetes and kidney failure. He physically lashed out at us if he thought we were looking at him 'peculiar-like' – which Ursula started to do as a matter of principle. I wasn't as brave and took to thinking of the ex-soldier as a trained killer, who might do me a nasty. I overlooked the reality that he couldn't spear a cooked potato with a dinner fork, let alone run me through with a bayonet.

With the huge emphasis placed on cleaning everything within two hundred miles of a patient, I remained on intimate terms with disinfectant and commodes, the bath, metal trolleys, patients' lockers, IV stands, bed frames, wheelchairs, the linen room and my new friends the clinical-room shelves.

After a while, there was nothing I didn't know about levers and castors and other parts that could fall off hospital equipment. Better still, thanks to mechanical skills inherited from my mother, I knew how to put everything back together.

Mum must have had second sight when I was packing for London and she had dropped a wrench and a double-ended screwdriver into my suitcase. 'You never know when you're going to need these,' she had said, Britain's greatest living expert on what should be in a nurse's pocket.

'Oh, for goodness' sake, Mum,' I'd remonstrated. 'It's a hospital, not a lawnmower-repair shop.' No way was I ever telling her how useful the tools were.

It was my third week on the ward when Sister Morag emerged from her office starving for game like a bear in springtime. And I was her quarry. Suddenly my list of things to clean expanded to include human bottoms, and I was thrown into a never-ending cycle of toileting patients, wiping bottoms and changing sheets covered with bodily fluids and excreta. And you know what? I didn't mind. Oh, it was ghastly all right, but I was caring for people, and that meant a great deal to me. What did bother me was that I still wasn't learning anything. After all, I'd been wiping my own bottom for a fair few years and had the process down pretty much perfect.

Refusing to fall by the wayside, I worked hard and complained little, a gargantuan achievement considering I still had my usual equipment-cleaning duties, an activity that dictated I was always late off duty. As Rosie kept telling me, I just had to get on with it. After all, I was doing real nursing care at last, albeit only at the business end.

'Have you taken a blood pressure yet or given an injection?' Fenella asked me one afternoon, when she was helping a patient drink tea from a feeder cup and I was wiping the same patient's locker.

'Nope. I haven't really done anything we learned in PTS,' I told her, and then added, 'Actually, Fenella, I don't remember how to take a blood pressure.'

'Oh dear,' she said, looking embarrassed.

'Oh dear is right,' I said rather icily, unable to hide my annoyance that she was allowed to do more proper nursing than me.

Mr Clegg was being kept as comfortable as possible with full nursing care, oxygen via a mask for when he was breathless, gentle ambulation, and medications to reduce his fluid retention and strengthen his heart function. He wasn't expected to live long, and I badly wanted to look after him, but all I did was smile each time I passed his bed. It wasn't nearly enough.

Then I had a great idea.

Nestled in the heart of the maze of buildings and link-corridors at St Giles was a peaceful grass quad-rangle open to the sky. Often, as I walked across the lawn, I thought about the workhouse history and won-dered who was beneath my feet, but today I dismissed such thoughts. I was in search of a public telephone.

I found one at the bottom of the stairs that led from the quadrangle up to St Giles nurses' home, and I telephoned Mrs Clegg, who enthusiastically agreed to my idea. Now all I had to do was wait until Saturday, Sister Morag's next day off, which took for ever to arrive.

At noon on Saturday, when Staff Nurse Tubby was at lunch, Klaus helped me lift Mr Clegg into a wheelchair and cover him with blankets that I had warmed on a radiator.

After checking the coast was clear, Klaus pushed Mr Clegg out to the quadrangle, with me alongside, pulling the large black oxygen cylinder that was attached by a tube to Mr Clegg's face mask. The weather was on our side: not too chilly and no rain or wind.

Carefully I removed the oxygen mask from Mr Clegg's face.

'Oh, my.' He murmured when he saw Mrs Clegg standing on the lawn with his beloved wire-haired fox terrier. Feebly he waved his hands and breathlessly called, 'Monty!'

Realizing who was under the blankets, Monty yelped excitedly. Mrs Clegg let the dog off the lead and he scampered over to Mr Clegg and jumped lightly on to his lap. It was a memorable moment: Mr Clegg hugging Monty and enjoying a Pal-scented facial, Mrs Clegg and Klaus smiling with pleasure, and me watching with a lump in my throat.

Mrs Clegg produced a red ball, and Monty jumped on to the grass and uttered a playful woof.

As Mr Clegg was too weak, I threw the ball, and Monty raced around the lawn after it, much to his master's delight.

Then everything went pear-shaped. Big-time.

'Johnson!' a voice screeched from above.

I looked up to see a furious-faced Sister Morag leaning out of a second-floor window in the nurses' home. Really, how was I supposed to know she lived there?

Sister Morag went ballistic, shouting that whoever was responsible for such a gross abuse of the rules would be sent to the director of nurse education, Sister Caroline, for possible dismissal.

Naturally, I did the first thing that came into my head and pointed straight at Klaus. I expect he still laughs about it . . .

It didn't matter whether the latest edict from the Royal College of Nursing was that the most senior nurse should be called chief nursing officer, director of nursing, number ten or simply matron: in hospitals the length and breadth of Britain, matrons reigned supreme. Single-handedly they could have stopped the Four Horsemen of the Apocalypse, and when it came to authority, in every area of hospital administration, matrons wielded power and commanded respect like no other. They worked hard and knew the name and diagnosis of every patient on their wards; the welfare of their charges and the good name of the hospital were their reasons for being.

What we didn't know was that, over the next decade, while cleverly giving the impression of doing the exact opposite, professional restructuring within nursing ranks and truckloads of new policies would slowly erode a matron's authority until people were in charge of hospitals who didn't know a thermometer from a chopstick.

On Dickens, whoever had the drug-trolley keys attached to their uniform was considered in charge and, when she was on duty, the Grand Poobah was Sister Morag.

Next in the pecking order were two staff nurses (both state registered nurses – SRNs), followed by third-year student nurses (one of whom was Ursula) and three state enrolled nurses (SENs completed a shorter, two-year training). There were several second-year student nurses (including Rosie), then Fenella and me, and last, two male ward orderlies, Klaus the German conchie and Guitano, an Italian Lothario, who was sleeping his way through the South London postcodes.

Three duties (or shifts) had to be covered – early, late and night duty – as well as days off and holidays. Apart from Staff Nurse Tubby, the second staff nurse (Typhoid Mary, as Rosie called her) was always off sick with a 'tummy bug', and we frequently had the company of a hard-working West Indian agency staff nurse called Gladness, a well-named peach of a lady. Gladness sang songs by Diana Ross and the Supremes as she worked, smiled at everyone, and wagged a pointy finger at patients who needed a good telling-off.

Apart from patient charts at the end of beds, there was scant paperwork on the ward that I could see. Stores and pharmacy request forms were completed by a staff nurse, meals were ordered by a student nurse, and before each duty changeover a nurse would sit at the nurses' desk in the middle of the ward and write notes in the Kardex – a metal flip file of lined cards on which were recorded each patient's current condition and what had happened during the shift. Doctors wrote what appeared to be hieroglyphics in patients' hospital notes, and these were filed in the trolley next to the nurses' desk ready to be pushed along on ward rounds.

Among the nurses, our other means of communication was a pretty old-fashioned concept known as 'talking', which we mostly did in hushed tones, as it was considered that if we had time to talk we were not working hard enough. Similar to the no make-up policy and no marriage policy, this was a logic that defied merit.

Morning, noon and night, one nurse was *allowed* to talk. With the rest of us huddled around the nurses' desk, a nurse from the earlier shift would flip through the aforementioned Kardex and read the latest entries aloud for 'report'. This provided a continual sharing of information on each patient's diagnosis, test results and specific care. I remember thinking: *One day I will write in the Kardex and flip over the pages and read aloud what I have written, and everyone will listen to me.* You can't argue with that sort of ambition, can you?

The cleaning workload on Dickens was heavy, and although I tried not to focus on it too much, I knew that other girls in my set were changing the occasional dirty sheets but were also practising tasks we had learned in PTS, all under the watchful eye of a ward sister or senior nurse.

For sure, someone at the top thought I was unsuitable to the calling, and I was certain that Sister

Morag was on notice to report my every mistake. She had quickly learned that I was responsible for the dog-in-the-quadrangle incident, and I was scheduled to see Sister Caroline for 'possible dismissal'. It was a black cloud hanging over my head, and I tried hard not to make any more mistakes.

There was relative safety for me in being at the arse-end of things, so to speak, but I worried that I was missing out on valuable learning opportunities. Unsure what to do about the situation, I watched enviously as other nurses moved about the ward (the *Benny Hill* theme tune wouldn't go amiss here), conducting the daily procedures of geriatric care: dressing leg ulcers; turning bedridden patients from side to side to prevent pressure sores; monitoring oxygen therapy; helping old men in and out of their pyjamas; lifting patients out of beds and into armchairs; making beds; handing out medications; balancing fluid charts; cleaning false teeth; feeding meals; answering phones; writing up notes – all of the things I wasn't allowed to do. Even Klaus and Guitano helped with bed-baths and general baths, and sometimes wheeled the men outside for a smoke.

I enjoyed working with Klaus, as he would help me clean in the afternoon if the ward was quiet, but I avoided Guitano. All female nurses did. He had wandering palmitis and passed too close at times, his hand or arm brushing against our breasts. It was creepy but clever, as I was unable to identify one definitive occasion that could not have been explained as an accident.

In the end, a spot of fisticuffs resolved the Guitano problem. He made the mistake of applying a bit of rear frottage action to Ursula in the linen cupboard, an incident she duly reported to her boyfriend, Jack. One evening, after a late duty, Jack (a rugby forward) waited for the offender outside the hospital gates.

'Guitano won't be picking his nose for a while,' Ursula happily reported to me the following day. 'Or touching our boobs again, Maggie.' I was happy too, but slightly peeved I hadn't resolved the issue myself.

We had one and a half days off a week, and the lower down the ladder we were the less likely it was that our day off would be at the weekend. In PTS, we were told that a thoughtful sister would roster us on a half-day before our day off and allow us to return on a late duty the following day, effectively giving us two days off. Without fail, Sister Morag rostered me on an early after my day off, which made going home to Fareham difficult. When I complained to Rosie about this, she informed me that there was nothing I could do and I just had to get on with it, but she said that about everything.

Then one day Rosie surprised me. I was telling her about the dog incident and how I was to see Sister Caroline, and that I was sure the hospital authorities were hoping I would make a mistake so they could throw me out.

'Have you got rocks in your head?' Rosie exclaimed in a loud voice. 'They don't want to get rid of you! Good Lord, Maggie, they need you! All student nurses have to work on geriatric wards in the group hospitals. Otherwise they'd never be able to afford to staff the hospitals!' Rosie was the maddest I had ever seen her.

'But I'm not learning anything,' I bleated, and then out it all came, with tears and a runny nose. 'I'm supposed to be a student learning to be a state registered nurse,' I wailed, 'but all I'm doing is menial work and I'm not even being paid for it! It's not training! It's just cleaning!'

Aware that I was slightly hysterical and we were both

talking in exclamation marks, I stopped blubbering, wiped my eyes and blew my nose.

Hopeless at maintaining rage, Rosie mellowed and put a hand on my shoulder. 'I know,' she said, finally sounding sympathetic. 'But it's how it's always been, Maggie. A lot of the time, student nurses are just cheap labour, and there is nothing we can do about it.'

'But at least you're nursing patients.'

'Basic nursing care,' Rosie said. 'I don't need to keep doing it to learn it. I'm not practising procedures I learned in my last school block. With the new technology on the wards, new drugs, new cardiac care and the changes in post-operative nursing, not to mention new transplant surgery, I should be practising those things. Actually, I've done so much geriatrics I'm worried I won't know the right things when I take my finals.'

Stunned by her admission, I was about to ask why she didn't complain but knew I would be told there was no point, so I took a different tack. 'Why don't kippers complain?' I asked. ('Kippers' were third-year student nurses, named after their tall hat, which was called a kipper, I think because it looked like a kipper when it was starched and pressed flat. Accordingly, first-year students were called 'paper caps', and second-year students 'frillies', due to their frilly headwear, which was slightly silly but not quite as ridiculous as the kipper.)

Rosie thought for a minute. 'Kippers have nearly finished their training. They don't want to rock the boat. They just want to qualify.'

'So we just get on with it, do we?'

'Yes, if you want a good ward report,' Rosie said.

A short time later, I was scrubbing a commode chair that we used to wheel patients in and out of the toilets when Gladness came into the bathroom. Hopelessly out of tune, she was singing what sounded like a Marvin Gaye song. Smiling at me, she stopped singing and said, 'I couldn't help overhearin' your . . . err . . . discussion with Nurse Rosie.' The soft cadence of her Jamaican accent radiated friendly warmth. 'Are you feeling better?'

I looked over my shoulder at her. 'Yes, thanks. I just have to get on with it, like Rosie says.'

Gladness perched her large bottom on the edge of the bath. 'You know,' she said, 'you might speak to your tutor. For what it's worth, not all ward sisters are like Morag. She thrives on dominating and belittling junior staff, but you are supposed to be a student, and I think you should be taking observations, feeding patients and tagging along on drug rounds.'

I stopped what I was doing and turned to face her. 'You do?'

'Yes, I do. At this early stage, in addition to basic nursing care of elderly patients, you should already be practising what you learned in PTS. There's a lot of training to cover in three years and you need to start now.'

'Okay, then,' I said, half smiling at her.

'Okay, then,' Gladness repeated, and gave me a nod of approval.

Launching herself upright, she affectionately patted my arm, then waddled back on to the ward, her behind swinging from side to side like two watermelons in a pillowcase.

After some thought, I decided to inform Sister Caroline of the cleaning situation and lack of supervision when I went to see her about the dog.

It was better than doing nothing.

Or maybe not.

CHAPTER 5

A Rebel with a Cause

St Giles Hospital, London: December 1970

A PROFESSIONAL APPROACH was important, and I prepared a speech before seeing Sister Caroline. She needed to know that I was aware I had been sent to Dickens not to test my mettle but as part of the hospital's cunning plan to staff geriatric wards with cheap, efficient labour. After apologizing about the dog, I would advise her that an economic crime was being committed right under her nose, and that management of the hospital budget was being placed ahead of clinical nurse training and tuition. The deception, I would go on to explain, was cleverly camouflaged by terms such as 'calling' and 'vocation', and I would add that the National Health Service knew full well the fiscal advantage in their subterfuge. I would also tell Sister Caroline that I was forbidden to marry because the authorities knew there wasn't a man on earth who would sanction such overt financial abuse of his wife.

The meeting went something like this.

I faced Sister Caroline across her desk, ready to be reprimanded about the dog. Out of the office window,

I could see hospital rooftops and gathering dark clouds – an ominous portent.

But Sister Caroline didn't appear cross. 'How are you enjoying your training, Nurse Johnson?' she asked, smiling warmly.

'Everything's wrong!' I blurted out, as my meticulously planned speech spun off into another vortex. 'The ward cleaner is paid a proper wage, and I'm doing more cleaning than her and I'm only paid a pittance!'

Aware that I had missed the point, I watched with angst as a frown formed across Sister Caroline's brow. So help me, I couldn't think of a single thing to say that would make more sense of my outburst. I waited for her to say, 'Stiff cheese!' but she didn't.

Slowly, Sister Caroline nodded, I think more to herself than to me. She put down her pen and sat back in her chair. 'What I'm hearing is that you don't like cleaning. Is that right?' she ventured.

'I don't dislike cleaning,' I explained, back in control, 'but it's all I'm doing. I'm supposed to be a student learning to be a state registered nurse, not a student learning to be a cleaner. I already know how to clean.'

She uttered a small laugh. 'I'm sure at times it seems like cleaning is all you are doing.'

'No,' I pressed, 'it really is mostly what I'm doing.'

Sister Caroline looked thoughtful for a while. Finally she said, 'There are many areas of nursing, and cleaning equipment is very important to minimize infection in the hospital. I'm afraid we all have to clean, Nurse Johnson, and we all have to start at the bottom.' She sat forward and placed her clasped hands on the desk as if to reinforce her remark. She also tried to look stern, but with such a serene face she couldn't carry it off.

Realizing that further explanation was required, I added: 'On other wards, nurses share the cleaning in the afternoons when patients are resting, or during visiting hours. I clean from the moment I arrive on the ward. I haven't taken a temperature yet. Or performed a complete bed-bath. Or taken a blood pressure.'

Sister Caroline's eyebrows shot up. 'Not even once?'

Doubting she believed me, I shook my head. 'I've bathed a tramp, given an unnecessary partial bed-bath, changed dirty beds and cleaned things. That's it. And my only supervision is from other students.'

My eyes were watering and I breathed in deeply to stave off approaching tears. 'I don't mind cleaning, really I don't,' I bleated, 'and I'm not afraid of hard work, but I want to be a good state registered nurse, and I can't if I'm not allowed to practise what I've learned in school.' Then my emotions got the better of me and I burst into tears.

Sister Caroline passed me a tissue and made notes while I brought my blubbering under control. When I had recovered, she asked, 'Are you on duty this Friday morning?'

'Yes, an early.' I sniffed and scrunched the wet tissue in my hand, not knowing what to do with it.

'I will ask Sister Bronwyn to join you and oversee your practical work.'

'But—' I started, anxious that I might be tested on something I hadn't practised.

'Yes, I know,' Sister Caroline interrupted, holding up her hand to stop further discussion. 'I have made a note that you haven't practised anything you learned in PTS. On Friday, Sister Bronwyn will assist you with some basic nursing care.'

Stunned that someone in authority had listened to me, I said, 'Thank you, Sister Caroline.'

She would, I felt sure, pull out all the stops to ensure that her students received a proper training, but that didn't make what was happening to me and many others right, and I like to think that Sister Caroline knew it.

Later in my training, I would discover that my complaint to Sister Caroline had not been misguided. Concerned nurses at the Royal College of Nursing were already successfully pressuring the government to review the quality and nature of professional training required for nurses and midwives. The review, to be undertaken by the historian Professor Asa Briggs (and called the Briggs Report), would be published in 1972, and would turn accepted training practice on its ear. It would also cause fiscal hearts at the Treasury to flutter nervously.

'A word of advice,' Sister Caroline offered, as I stood up to leave. 'Inform Sister Morag that Sister Bronwyn will be working with you on Friday.'

I nodded. 'I will, thank you.'

Glancing out of the window, I noticed the dark skies had passed and there were patches of blue peeking through fluffy white clouds. Enough blue, as my Nana Higgins used to say, to patch a sailor's breeches.

I was halfway down the stairs when I realized that Sister Caroline hadn't mentioned the dog.

It was Friday morning and I was scrubbing the bath on Dickens when Sister Bronwyn and a frosty-faced Sister Morag walked into the bathroom. The room was icy cold as I had opened the windows to disperse the smell of disinfectant. Both sisters shuddered and folded their arms for warmth.

'Why didn't you inform me a tutor was coming today?' Sister Morag demanded. 'This is most inconvenient.'

Without waiting for an answer, she stuck her nose into the air and flounced out of the bathroom. 'And shut those windows!' she barked over her shoulder.

'Yes, why didn't you tell Sister Morag?' Sister Bronwyn asked. Her tone was more questioning than reprimanding.

'Because I was scared she would make a liar of me and I'd be taking temperatures when you arrived,' I answered bravely. Student nurses simply didn't speak to sisters like that, but I felt I had nothing to lose.

'That's ridiculous!' she exclaimed.

'Yes, it is,' I countered. 'I'm sorry, but it's true.'

Sister Bronwyn didn't reply. Aware of her surveillance while I leaned over and rinsed the bath, I wondered if, like me, she was questioning how a tutor coming to the ward could be inconvenient. It was, after all, an extra pair of hands.

'We will start with observations,' she said, when I was ready. 'I will do the first set and show you how to mark the patient's chart, and you will do the rest.' Then she paused and her face softened. 'And I will help you.'

It was a welcome olive branch, and I acknowledged it with a smile. We washed our hands and I followed her on to the ward. Neither of us closed the windows.

Our first patient was Mr Barlow. He scowled menacingly at me while I explained to Sister Bronwyn that his diagnosis was rheumatoid arthritis, and that he was having respite care while his wife underwent surgery.

Reaching up, Sister Bronwyn removed the thermometer from the wall holder above Mr Barlow's bed. Grasping it firmly between her thumb and forefinger, she flicked her wrist a few times, which made a supremely professional nursing sound, then checked that the mercury level measured below normal body temperature. After popping the thermometer under Mr Barlow's tongue, she placed three fingers on his radial pulse and lifted the fob watch pinned to her chest. Aloud, she counted the pulse beats for a minute. Then she counted his respirations for another minute. Removing the thermometer from his mouth, she checked the mercury level.

'Perfectly normal,' she announced.

'What ya bleedin' expect?' Mr Barlow grumbled. 'I shouldn't be in 'ere.'

'I'm sure there are some who wish you weren't,' Sister Bronwyn replied curtly, pushed up his pyjama sleeve, and opened the wooden box containing the sphygmomanometer. She wrapped the cuff around his right arm, then with practised efficiency put the stethoscope into her ears and pumped up the cuff until the Velcro started to crackle.

'Err . . . watch it . . . that 'urts!' Mr Barlow complained loudly. I was having a hard time not sniggering. This was fine sport.

Sister Bronwyn placed the end of the stethoscope on Mr Barlow's brachial pulse, on the inside of his elbow, and slowly released the valve on the pump. She indicated for me to watch the mercury level descend on the sphygmomanometer.

'A hundred and ninety over a hundred. Your blood pressure is high, Mr Bartlett,' she said. 'Nurse Johnson and I will inform Sister Morag.'

'The name's Barlow, ya dozy cow.' Snorting, he spat into the kidney dish beside his bed and wiped his mouth with his pyjama sleeve.

Ignoring him, Sister Bronwyn released the valve completely, removed the cuff and showed me how to record the observations on the chart that hung at the end of the bed.

'On rare occasions,' she said, in a hushed voice, 'patients can be very ill-tempered and the nurse must ignore their bad behaviour.'

Rare occasions? Where had this woman been?

The next patient was Mr Hyde, and out of sheer naughtiness I looked at him peculiar-like. It achieved the desired result, and he went off like a rocket.

'Don't you look at me, you hairy old bat,' he threatened Sister Bronwyn. 'And you can bugger off an' all,' he shouted at me.

Unnerved, Sister Bronwyn whispered in my ear, 'I think we should move on.'

The next patient was Harry Lipton, who had lost both legs to gangrene from peripheral neuropathy, a complication of his diabetes. He received daily insulin injections, was on regular urine testing to assess his sugar levels and had a strict diet to control his hyperglycaemic attacks. Mr Lipton was a rag-and-bone man and, according to the night nurses, he would call out, 'Rag and bone!' in his sleep. There was a metal frame in his bed to keep the sheets off his stumps, one of which was ulcerated and required daily dressings. He was an ill-tempered old cuss, more used to communicating with a horse than with people, but he was an angel compared with Mr Hyde.

Nervously I told Mr Lipton I was going to take his temperature. On the first flick of my wrist, the thermometer shot out of my hand, spun across the floor and broke. Mr Lipton laughed, and I blushed red as a pillar box as Sister Bronwyn and I chased small speeding balls of mercury around the floor. Rosie, bless her, appeared with a new thermometer. The second time, I was more successful, but when I removed the thermometer from Mr Lipton's mouth I couldn't see the mercury level for the life of me. Where was it? I twisted and turned the thermometer, but the silver line remained elusive. 'Normal,' I announced, hoping it was.

'You really haven't done observations before, have you?' Sister Bronwyn remarked.

I shook my head. 'No. I'm sorry.'

'It's not your fault, Nurse Johnson,' she said. 'Now, we have a lot to cover this morning, and I suggest we get on with it.'

Despite a lack of cooperation and a lot of bad language from patients, I managed the rest of the observations without further breakages, and I was pleasantly surprised when Sister Bronwyn commented on how well I was coping with the unusual hostility on the ward.

After a brief word with Sister Morag in her office, Sister Bronwyn returned and said, 'We are to give Mr Snape a bed-bath.'

My spirits sank. Of all the patients . . .

Glancing towards the office, I saw Sister Morag watching us. She was grinning like a cat with a mouthful of canary. Sister Bronwyn followed my gaze and asked, 'Why is Sister Morag smiling?'

'I think because Mr Snape is a very difficult patient,' I answered truthfully.

'We shall see about that!' Sister Bronwyn said decisively, and quick sticks we had a bowl of steaming hot water, towels, soap, and curtains pulled around his bed. Mr Snape was startled by this sudden flurry of activity about his person, and he sat rigid as a statue as we washed and dried him from top to toe. He didn't even say a word when Sister Bronwyn pulled back his foreskin and told me how important it was to keep that area clean. I, on the other hand, nearly passed out. Really, you couldn't make this stuff up.

Working together, we clipped our patient's nails, shaved his face, trimmed his eyebrows, brushed his hair and dressed him in clean pyjamas.

'There, ready for Crufts,' Sister Bronwyn announced. Unbelievably, Mr Snape laughed.

'Oh, I do miss my patients,' Sister Bronwyn said, and sighed. 'Do you like football, Mr Snape?'

'I'm a Pompey supporter,' he confirmed with a nod. His eyes were shining at the thought of his beloved Portsmouth. I couldn't believe it.

'Nurse Johnson will go to the main entrance for a newspaper with the football results,' she said.

'Right away, Sister,' I chirped, and hot-footed it to the main entrance. Returning five minutes later with a newspaper, I was amazed that Mr Snape hadn't lost his good humour.

'Thanks, love,' he said, as if we'd been friends for ages. Bemused, I smiled at him.

I worked hard for the rest of the morning, spurred

on by enjoyment. Sister Bronwyn and I completed two more bed-baths, filled in a patient's fluid chart and changed the sterile dressing on Mr Lipton's stump. I felt light-headed when I saw his wound, and Sister Bronwyn told me to take deep breaths and just get on with it, which made me chuckle.

Next we changed the oxygen cylinder beside Mr Clegg's bed, and it didn't explode as I had stupidly feared. Hearing us, Mr Clegg opened his eyes, pulled off his oxygen mask and told Sister Bronwyn that I had a heart of gold.

'Do you know what she did?' he puffed, his voice so faint that she had to lean forward to hear him. And before I could stop him, he told her about Monty's visit. 'She got into terrible trouble,' he said, before taking a big whiff of oxygen.

'Did she, indeed?' Sister Bronwyn remarked. I didn't dare look at her.

'Yes,' Mr Clegg said, removing his mask again. 'It's the best thing that's happened to me . . . seeing the missus and Monty like that.'

Closing my eyes, I wanted to run away and keep running until I reached Dover.

'She's a good nurse,' he managed.

'Not yet,' I heard Sister Bronwyn say, 'but she could be one day.'

Her voice sounded tinged with amusement. I opened my eyes and Sister Bronwyn was smiling at me.

I could have hugged her. And Mr Clegg.

During my remaining weeks on Dickens Sister Morag made my life a living hell. This she achieved by allocating to me every unsavoury job that concerned matters lavatorial, and by sending me out into the cold to retrieve imaginary spectacles, watches and false teeth that she was *certain* were in the slops bin behind the kitchen. She also falsely accused me of losing a pair of expensive Spencer Wells forceps and tried unsuccessfully to have the hospital dock the replacement cost from my allowance.

Two weeks before Christmas most of my friends and I were moved from our shared rooms at Hambledon House to our own rooms at St Giles nurses' home. Thrilled, I set about decorating my room the Maggie way, starting with the strategic placement of my lava lamp beside the bed. On my first free day, I caught a bus to Habitat on Tottenham Court Road and purchased six green Casa Pupo mugs, a teapot, a navy-blue beanbag, a red vase and a stuffed hedgehog. I bought Aubrey Beardsley and Toulouse-Lautrec posters at a shop in Piccadilly Circus, and two paisley-print tablecloths in Carnaby Street. I used one as a bedspread and draped the other across a wall for a harem effect. I also hung my copy of 'Desiderata' above my bed in case I needed to go placidly amid the noise and haste.

In no time at all I had the place looking very *House and Garden*. Visitors could sit on the beanbag and read 'Desiderata' while I brewed tea, and then we could both listen to Simon and Garfunkel on my reel-to-reel tape recorder. It was perfect, although any excitement gained by having a room of my own was tempered by the fact that I was two doors up from Sister Morag.

Mr Clegg died a few days before Christmas. Knowing I was fond of him, Rosie came to my room and told me that he had died peacefully, and that she and Ursula had performed the last offices. Rosie talked me out of attending his funeral by saying that if I started that nonsense now, I would be attending funerals on my days off for the next three years.

'But he was special,' I insisted.

'They're all special,' Rosie replied. 'That's the whole point.'

Before going on annual leave at Christmas, Sister Morag wrote me a stinker of a ward report. She also rostered me to work over Christmas, thereby scuppering any plans of a Johnson family celebration. It must have been a great disappointment to her when I wasn't as bothered as she might have hoped. You see, I had heard that Christmas on the wards could be a lot of fun and I was looking forward to seeing if it was true, although exactly how much fun it could be on Dickens with the cast of Dante's *Inferno* remained to be seen.

After I finished my late duty on Christmas Eve, Jan, Laurel and I kicked off the two-day event with a couple of gin and tonics, then trotted across the road to St Giles Church for midnight mass. I wasn't keen on the church idea as it was freezing outside, but I didn't want to be alone, so I tagged along. A spooky old building, the church was the quintessential Gothic nightmare, with broken tombs, creaky gates and a hooting owl.

A first-timer for midnight mass, indeed a first-timer for any religious service, I was overwhelmed by the soaring ceilings, the stained-glass windows, the glorious carol singing and the infectious joy that bounced off the walls but, as Laurel pointed out, gin will do that to you if you've missed dinner.

Christmas Eve 1970 produced an unbelievable finale. In the early hours of Christmas morning, as we emerged from the church into the yellow glow from the street lights, it started to snow – perfect white crystals that drifted softly to the ground.

'It's just like Canada,' Laurel said excitedly. She turned her face upwards and opened her mouth to catch the flakes.

'Not quite as much snow, though,' Jan said, laughing.

It turned out to be true about Christmas in hospital. It was a lot of fun – for staff, anyway. With Sister Morag away, Tubby in Wales and Typhoid Mary off sick, we were a little short-staffed with only Ursula, Rosie, a new SEN called Paige and me, and it was a great relief when Gladness walked through the door and took charge. Wearing a Santa hat, she marched into the sister's office with a basket full of mince pies, red wine, Christmas cake and candied fruit.

'Right,' she said, rubbing her hands together. 'Let's get everyone washed and dressed and have some fun!'

Patients who were well enough to be discharged for a few days had gone home, and some were replaced by homeless men who could use two days in a warm bed and a bit of turkey. Veterans of the street, they had handed themselves in at the main entrance, and I was delighted to discover that One-Ear Jones was among them. Naturally he stank to high Heaven, was tanked to the eyeballs and didn't know Rosie or me from a bar of soap.

As we worked, we played Bing Crosby's 'White Christmas', sang carols, and every so often nipped into the office for a cup of tea and a mince pie. For lunch, there was turkey and all the trimmings, and during the afternoon visitors arrived with presents for their relatives and chocolates for us. Nurses and doctors who were on duty visited all the wards to share a toast, and Gladness's husband, Horatio, and her four children arrived with more chocolates. If only every day could be like that.

After Christmas I learned that in mid-January Fenella and I would start on Fisk and Cheere, the two ear, nose and throat (ENT) wards at King's. I was disappointed that I would still be with Fenella. Anyone could see that she was an excellent student nurse – obedient, hard-working and diligent – and I couldn't help feeling a little in her shadow. Nevertheless, I was thrilled about King's and started counting the days.

The realization that I had shown endurance in finishing my time on Dickens had given me a surprising feeling of power. Maybe I had a smattering of inner strength, and maybe, just maybe, things might be a little easier from now on.

Another good thing: the interminable cleaning had forced me to confront some of the profession's accepted norms that I believed to be wrong, namely the use of student nurses as cheap labour, and the lack of teaching and supervision on my ward. A rebel with a cause, I discovered that it was important for me to understand the reason why I was doing something rather than 'just getting on with it' because that was the way things had always been done.

So, look out Fisk and Cheere, here I come . . .

CHAPTER 6

The Great Paper Underpants Fiasco

King's College Hospital, London: January 1971

SOUND THE TRUMPETS! At last, the day had arrived when I was going to tread the hallowed floors of one of King's College Hospital's world-renowned wards. At least, they were world-renowned according to the sisters who had interviewed me. I didn't care if the wards were famous or not. The important thing for me was that I was finally going to have me a piece of that exceptional clinical nurse training I had heard so much about.

In honour of the occasion, I was brushing a little brown mascara on to my eyelashes. As another act of insubordination, I was wearing Janet Reger undies beneath my neatly pressed uniform; no one would know about the undies, but if anyone spotted the make-up, I would be off to the gulag.

Even Jan, our champion darer, was sceptical I could get away with it. Still in her pyjamas, and sitting with her feet up on my bed at St Giles nurses' home, she was drinking coffee and flicking through my

Toohey's Medicine for Nurses, pretending not to be nervous about her first day on an acute male medical ward at Dulwich Hospital. Jan now lived in the nurses' home at Dulwich Hospital and had stayed over last night in a spare room at St Giles.

'Make sure your passport is up to date so they can send you to Russia,' she advised drily, as I recklessly dusted blusher on to my cheeks.

'You know why I'm doing this,' I said, screwing up my nose in her direction.

'No one notices it, Maggie, and anyway, it adds character to your face.' She sighed loudly and closed the book. 'I'll never grasp the endocrine system as long as I live.'

Ignoring her, I dabbed foundation on the ugly scar above my right cheekbone. Thicker in the middle, it resembled the mouth on a smiley face, the dark colouring obvious against my pale skin.

It was a childhood accident that had caused the damage. Three years old, I had fallen off a tricycle that was doubling as a horse. As well as fracturing my skull, I had taken a good chunk of flesh out of the side of my face and destroyed a perfectly lovely display of lobelia.

The lobelia was replanted, and my head was put back together by doctors in Portsmouth. The resultant scar was amateur and pronounced, and my brother never tired of telling me that it could be seen by passengers from overhead aircraft.

'Golly, look at the time,' Jan shrieked in alarm. Leaping up, she plonked her mug on my bedside table and raced back to the spare room to get dressed.

I peered out of the window. It was six thirty in the wintry pre-dawn, black as pitch outside, raining, and so windy that raindrops were tadpoling up the windowpane as well as down. Fraser was driving Adele, Miranda and Kathy in his Ford Anglia to their wards at St Francis. I wondered how they would fare. Each had shown sympathy to my bleating about Dickens, but I knew they hadn't believed the full horror of it.

Polly was starting on a men's surgical ward here at St Giles, and Meredith and Laurel were starting on a women's surgical ward also at St Giles. Tilly, who was supposed to be on a medical ward at King's, was in bed with influenza.

Jan and I would be taking the hospital transport that ferried nurses from the various nurses' homes to group hospitals in the early morning. I put on my coat and hat and grabbed my umbrella.

I entered King's College Hospital via the nurses'-home door and collected a key to a locker. Trembling – which I blamed on the weather – I hung up my coat and hat and put on my paper cap and a crisp new apron, ready for action.

Managed as one unit, the two ENT wards, Fisk and Cheere, were opposite each other at the end of the main corridor on the first floor at King's, males on Fisk and females on Cheere. In between were the kitchen, a clinical room, utility rooms and Sister Marybeth's office. Awestruck by the modern magnificence of it all, I stood in the office with fourteen other nurses, including Sister Marybeth, and listened to morning report from the night nurses. Fenella was also on her first day and looked decidedly nervous. I gave her a reassuring smile.

Apart from the fact that the patients mentioned were admitted for treatment to improve or cure their primary diagnosis, and were all expected to be discharged home, the other thing that made this report so spectacularly different from Dickens was the presence of a male staff nurse. I had not seen a male staff nurse before, and he was a curiosity that deserved my thorough inspection. Wearing a white tunic over trousers, he was short for a man and nuggetty thick. Strong as a bull, I imagined. His name was Staff Nurse Hutchins, and I wondered if he would be called Mister Sister on his next promotion.

Aware of my scrutiny, his friendly face broke into a smile and he winked at me. Blushing, I fixed my stare on the night nurse and paid attention to her report, marvelling over the incredible words: septoplasty, stapedectomy, tympanoplasty and cholesteatoma. Thrilling stuff, and way better than *Dr Finlay's Casebook*.

My eyes wandered to Sister Marybeth. A handsome, middle-aged woman with short, iron-grey hair, she wore a permanent smile that was a little cool around the edges. When report was finished, she thanked the night nurse and rolled up her sleeves. Surely she wasn't going to work on the ward?

Oh yes she was! With no-nonsense efficiency, Sister Marybeth allocated the workload, tasking Staff Nurse Hutchins to supervise Fenella on Cheere, and when only two of us remained, she stood up and said, 'Come along, Johnson.'

I followed her to the kitchen, where we prepared a vat of porridge large enough to feed France. Thanks to my mother, I was intimately acquainted with porridge, and I worked with confidence, aware of the coolish smile that said, *I'm nice, but not too nice.*

'On the ward, don't do anything you're unsure of,' Sister Marybeth said, handing me the salt. 'Always ask a senior nurse.'

Worried our close proximity would expose my make-up, I added salt and stirred the porridge with an outstretched arm – an unusual catering practice she might not have seen before.

'No one's going to shoot you for asking questions,' she went on, 'and if you develop a sore throat, call in sick and have a throat swab taken. Many of our patients have throat surgery and we must be careful.'

Leaving the porridge on low, we left the kitchen and I was told to work with Staff Nurse Julia Carter on Fisk. 'You can't miss her,' Sister said jovially. 'Look where all the men are looking and you'll find her.'

They were good directions. With a figure to die for, cornflower-blue eyes and hair the colour of windswept wheat, nature had been kind to Staff Nurse Carter, but she didn't look too happy at having a paper cap on her hands. Although she was only a few years older than me, Victorian standards were maintained and we addressed each other formally.

'We have five men for theatre, Johnson,' she said. 'We will be prepping them for surgery.'

I could hardly wait. 'Do we stay on the male side all day?' I enquired, keen with the questions.

'Mostly, yes, but we cross to Cheere delivering breakfast, and if there's an emergency or if Sister wants us to special a patient.'

'What's "special"?' I asked. I had no idea.

She regarded me strangely, as if the answer was obvious. Finally realizing I didn't have a clue, she said, 'It's when one nurse stays with a patient to monitor their vital signs and provide constant critical care. I'm surprised you don't know that.'

Asking questions might not be the go here, I told myself.

The large breakfast trolley containing shelves of breakfast trays arrived and I went to the kitchen and loaded the porridge, bowls, spoons, milk and brown sugar on to a small kitchen trolley and wheeled it out on to Cheere. Maggie, *chef magnifique.*

Both Fisk and Cheere were of traditional pavilion ward design, otherwise called Nightingale wards. Long, narrow and flooded with daylight, they had high ceilings and tall windows between each of the iron-frame beds that lined the walls. The windows opened at the top and provided welcome cross-ventilation in summer. For now, winter warmth was courtesy of a large heater in the centre of the ward, next to the nurses' desk.

Avoiding patients with NBM (nil by mouth) signs over their beds, I ladled porridge into bowls, added milk and sugar as requested, and everyone thanked me. The atmosphere was light years away from the unhappy environment of Dickens.

Fifteen minutes later, I was in the clinical room attempting to draw up a pre-med injection of Omnopon and scopolamine for Gavin Harefield, aged twenty, a second-year St George's medical student whose nose had been seriously rearranged during an inter-hospital rugby match. Listed to have a rhinoplasty (repair of broken nose), he would be having his pre-med an hour before theatre to relax him prior to anaesthetic.

'Don't you know how to break the top off an ampoule, Johnson?' Staff Nurse Carter said, obviously irritated.

'No, I don't,' I replied glumly, and stared at the glass ampoule in my hand.

Incredulous, she asked, 'Where have you been since last September? Outer Mongolia?'

'Dickens at St Giles.'

'Not Sister Morag?'

I nodded solemnly. 'Yes.'

'How dreadful!' she exclaimed. Just like that her manner changed: she smiled and touched my arm. 'Here, let me show you how to do it.'

With new-found patience, Carter demonstrated how to flick the ampoule to transfer the fluid into the base, snap the glass at the neck, then attach a needle to the syringe and draw up the fluid. It took three attempts, a dropped syringe and a bloody finger (mine) for me to grasp the process.

'Have you given an injection?' she asked, when the pre-med was ready.

I shook my head. Oh, help. I didn't want my first injection to be on a medical student.

'Come on, Johnson,' she said. 'No time like the present. And call him Gavin – he'll feel more comfortable.'

As nervous as a prisoner going to the gallows, albeit with a strange enthusiasm for the upcoming activity, I followed her on to the ward, a happening place with nurses tending patients, doctors reading notes, phones ringing, machines rumbling and cleaners mopping. A few patients were playing cards near the heater, and others with bandages wrapped around their heads were lying on beds. A good number had black eyes and dressings across their noses. Every single man watched Staff Nurse Carter walk past. Including the doctors.

'Gavin Harefield?' Carter asked the patient lying on bed fourteen, as she pulled the curtains.

'That's me,' he said, with a nasal twang. He was a fit-looking young man with longish dark hair and a nose that resembled a champagne cork.

Smiling reassuringly, Carter and I checked his wristband, the medication chart and his consent form for the operation. Crikey, this was brilliant. I was actually checking something. I couldn't wait to tell everyone.

'Are you allergic to anything, Gavin?' Carter asked him.

'No.'

'Have you passed urine recently?'

'Just now. Another nurse tested it.'

Carter examined the sheet of paper and nodded. 'Has the anaesthetist been?'

'I don't know, you'll have to ask him.'

This elicited an impromptu laugh from me.

'An oldie, but a goodie,' Carter said, laughing softly. 'Has the anaesthetist been to see you?'

Gavin nodded. 'It sounds like I'm not going to be as pretty as you.'

'Your nose will be swollen,' Carter explained, ignoring his flattery. 'And you'll have gauze plugs in your nostrils to stop the bleeding, so you'll be breathing through your mouth. When you come round, you'll be brought back to us and I'll give you something for pain and to stop any nausea. We'll take good care of you, I promise. Any questions?'

Gavin bit his lip. 'Will one of you come to theatre and stay with me until I'm asleep?'

'Yes, of course,' Carter said, without hesitation. She took his hand and squeezed it. 'Now you'll have to do something for us. This is Johnson's first injection, and you are going to be a good chap and not move. Isn't that right?'

'I'm not scared of needles,' Gavin said. 'Just operations. Bit daft for a medical student, isn't it?'

'Being in the profession doesn't give you a pass key,' Carter told him.

I felt the heat of adrenalin course through my veins. Gavin turned on to his side and Carter pulled down his pyjama pants. 'Visually divide the buttock into four and aim for the upper outer quadrant,' she said. 'And never tell a patient it won't hurt. It's a lie, and they'll lose trust in you.'

Picking my target, I wiped Gavin's skin with an alcohol swab.

'Ouch!' he yelled.

'You rotten thing,' Carter admonished him. 'She hasn't done it yet!'

Taking the opportunity while he was laughing, I plunged the needle into his backside, fumbled a bit as I drew the plunger back to make sure I wasn't in a vein and, when no blood entered the syringe chamber, slowly squeezed the pre-med into his muscle. Removing the needle quickly, I wiped the area again with the swab.

'All done, Gavin,' I said proudly.

'I didn't feel a thing,' he said over his shoulder, although I knew it must have hurt.

'Johnson will be back to dress you for theatre,' Carter told him. 'You have to wear a gown and a paper hat to cover your hair. Any jewellery?'

Gavin shook his head.

'Back in a minute,' I said, thinking that no way would I be helping Gavin undress and put on the theatre garb. I'd die of embarrassment and so might he.

The Great Paper Underpants Fiasco

After all, no one would know I hadn't helped him. At least, that was what I thought when I collected a prepared theatre pile from the clinical room, took it to Gavin and left him to change.

Shadowed by Staff Nurse Carter, I completed four more pre-meds and surgical preps. The last pre-med done, Carter looked at her fob watch. 'Time to relieve Hastings for her break.'

We scrubbed our hands and walked to bed eight and seventy-year-old Rex Steadman, who had throat cancer. The tumour had been surgically removed and a tracheostomy – a surgical opening in his throat below the larynx – allowed him to breathe.

Nurse Hastings, a kipper, handed over to us. Hearing voices, Mr Steadman opened his eyes.

'Hello,' Carter said softly. 'I'm going to suction the mucus out of your throat and change the dressing.'

While I watched, Carter removed the bib that covered Mr Steadman's throat. There was an indwelling plastic tube in the opening to keep his airway clear, and a moist, bubbling noise as Mr Steadman breathed in and out. I tried unsuccessfully not to look shocked at the hole in the poor man's neck. It was very grown-up viewing.

'Watch closely,' Carter said. She switched on the suction machine, attached a clean tube, inserted the tubing into the tracheostomy hole, and gently rotated it to remove mucus build-up.

'Only use suction for five to ten seconds,' she said. 'Check the secretions are clear. We don't want to see blood or yellowy-green discharge, which could indicate infection. And we don't see either. You're doing fine, Mr Steadman.'

Carter supervised while I rinsed the suction tube

in sterile water, changed the IV infusion bottle of normal saline (a salt and water solution) and adjusted the drips. My hands were shaking but I managed not to drop anything. We sat Mr Steadman up and rearranged his pillows, gently cleaned his mouth, then changed the sterile dressing around the tracheostomy.

'You are looking for a clean wound, Johnson,' Carter instructed me, as she wiped around the tracheostomy, discarding each wipe after a single use. 'And this is a clean wound, Mr Steadman.'

Taking extreme care, and sensibly not letting me do it, Carter inserted gauze under the outside wings of the tracheostomy tube to prevent chafing. 'Can you swallow easily, Mr Steadman?' she asked. He gave a weak nod.

'Good,' she said. 'Tomorrow you'll be feeling brighter. I'll organize a pen and paper so you can communicate with us until the speech therapist visits you. We should probably tell Johnson that there is no air flowing over your vocal cords, so you can't talk.'

Mr Steadman gingerly turned his head towards me and managed a glimmer of a smile. Feeling overwhelmed by his helplessness and the immense trust he placed in us, I beamed my ten-megawatt smile back at him, the one usually reserved for my father.

'Time for you to take Gavin Harefield to theatre,' Carter said, when the theatre porter walked on to the ward. 'Off you trot.'

Oh, my goodness, what a buzz I felt walking beside Gavin's trolley as we wheeled him to theatre. A couple of visitors stared at me and I bestowed on them a curt nod. I was far too important to talk to them.

'Hello, I'm the anaesthetist, Dr Wolfbane,' a

cadaverous-looking man in theatre greens and white clogs said to me as we entered the anaesthetic room. He bore a strong resemblance to someone I had seen before, but I couldn't work out who.

'Is this Gavin Harefield?' he asked.

'Yes.' I passed over the notes and picked up Gavin's hand.

'You can go . . . Nurse Johnson,' Dr Wolfbane said, as he took a good long look at the name badge pinned to the top right-hand side of my apron bib, over my ample bosom.

'I'd rather stay,' I replied assertively, conscious of Gavin's request for me to remain. I was annoyed by the doctor's unnecessarily long examination of my name badge. He must have thought I was born yesterday.

'Okay,' Dr Wolfbane said, and he gave me a look that was half smile and half *I'm gonna get you*. I had seen that wolfish look on men before.

Perching on a stool, Wolfbane asked Gavin what operation he was having, inspected the notes and checked Gavin's wristband. 'All's good,' he muttered.

I kept hold of Gavin's hand while a butterfly needle was inserted into the back of his other hand. Then Wolfbane placed a mask over Gavin's face and said, 'Count backwards from ten.'

'Ten, nine . . .' I started.

'Not you,' Wolfbane said, casting his eyes upwards. 'I mean Gavin!'

Gavin counted to eight and his hand went weak. He was under.

My job done, I turned to leave.

'Don't go, Nurse Johnson,' Dr Wolfbane said. 'I want to ask you something.'

Oh, here we go, I thought. The bosoms are going to be asked out to dinner.

Audibly sighing, I asked, 'Yes, what is it?'

'You're new, aren't you?'

'Yes, so?' I answered flippantly.

'Well,' he said, 'is there a special reason your patient has paper underpants on his head?'

I looked at Gavin. Sure enough, he had a pair of paper underpants pulled over his hair. Blushing, I clamped my hand over my mouth and fled, Wolfbane's laughter ringing in my ears.

In a panic, I checked other patients I had prepped. Thankfully, each had a paper hat on his head. Where had the paper underpants come from? Had Gavin done it for a laugh? Either way, it would teach me to do as I was told and dress a patient for theatre.

Staff Nurse Carter saw me looking anxious and came over. 'Everything all right in theatre?' she asked.

'Yes, thanks,' I lied.

'Hello, Maggie,' a voice said, and I spun round. Kip was walking past in his white coat, one of an entourage of male medical students and male doctors following the male consultant towards Mr Steadman's bed (medicine was as testosterone-heavy as engineering, although females were making inroads into both professions).

Carter collected Mr Steadman's notes and indicated for me to follow her. She handed the notes to the ENT registrar, Dr Brown, a tallish man in his late thirties with dark, matinee-idol looks and a superior air. Registrars were hospital-based doctors who had served time as a houseman and were undertaking four to six years in a specialist field.

Nurse Hastings and I hung back out of the way. Catching Kip's eye, I grimaced at him. This was the first time we had seen each other in a ward situation and I was strangely uncomfortable with it. I sensed he was too. Both young, we were finding our feet with our youthful romance.

We stood in a sedate group while the consultant outlined to his entourage the effects of throat cancer, articulated the surgical process and explained how pleased he was that he had successfully removed all of the malignant growth from Mr Steadman's larynx.

This appeared to be news to Mr Steadman, and tears of what I assumed were emotional relief rolled down his cheeks. Carter rested her hand proprietorially on Mr Steadman's arm and looked crossly at the consultant. 'If you will excuse us,' she said tersely, then to me, 'Johnson, pull the curtains around the bed, please.'

Nonplussed by her brave doctor-bossing, I pulled the curtains and watched Carter perch on the bed and wipe Mr Steadman's eyes with a tissue. Then a hand came through the curtains and Nurse Hastings yanked me out. 'The poor man doesn't need an audience,' she censured.

'So now you know what nurses do, lads,' the consultant said, with a guilty grin. A middle-aged man with a receding hairline, he had the confidence of wealth and position and the clipped diction of a public-school education. 'They're like mother tigers with cubs when protecting their patients from a doctor's insensitivity!'

There was a brown-nosing display of required guffaws and then, as if the idea had just come to him, the consultant said, 'You know, chaps, doctors and nurses have different responsibilities.'

The medical students looked blank, and I could see the consultant's mind registering the need for further explanation. 'Doctors order tests,' he went on, 'and we make the diagnosis and medical decisions and do the cutting, but the patient's welfare, safety, care and the constant monitoring of their condition is the nurses' responsibility.'

He smiled at Hastings and me. 'I think we doctors need to be reminded of that occasionally.'

Hastings and I exchanged raised eyebrows, and a profound clarity suddenly revealed itself to me. The most important person in the doctor-nurse-patient triangle was the patient, and not, as I had thought, and as many others including the doctor *and* the patient still think, the doctor. It was a realization that would cement for me a solid understanding of the purpose of my profession as distinct from that of the medical profession. And for such a momentous revelation, it's odd that I can't recall the consultant's name.

When Mr Steadman had composed himself, Carter pulled back the curtains.

'I apologize, Mr Steadman,' the consultant said, with feeling. 'You're in good hands. I'll see you tomorrow.'

As Dr Brown handed the notes back to Carter, I caught the brief caress of his hand on her forearm. Kip saw it too and flashed me a wicked smile.

Doctors and nurses, eh? We were all at it!

Carter and I watched the consultant and his ducklings leave, and laughed out loud when he stopped to look at something and his students concertinaed into the back of him.

'I think Dr Brown is gorgeous,' Carter declared, as she put Mr Steadman's notes back in the trolley.

'He's not my type,' I said flatly, and she looked at me as if I was mad. Anyone with half a brain could see the man was hotter than vindaloo.

The rest of the day was filled with new experiences. Supervised by Julia (who by mid-afternoon had decided we could drop the formalities), I removed gauze plugs from the nostrils of a man who'd had a deviated septum repaired, and learned how to syringe wax out of impacted ears. And, take it from me, you wouldn't want to do that last exercise before dinner.

There was no end to the breadth of my afternoon education. Julia confirmed that she and Dr Brown were playing doctors and nurses off duty, and that Brown had vowed to leave his wife, who didn't understand him. How men got away with such nonsense was beyond me. And why intelligent women believed them. I decided to lend Julia *The Female Eunuch*. Maybe that would knock some sense into her.

At the end of my duty, I went to Sister's office to ask if I could leave.

'Did you enjoy your first day on Fisk?' she asked.

'I loved it!' I burst out.

'Good. I'm keeping you on the same duties as Carter. She tells me you need to catch up with basic tasks.'

Whingeing never scored Brownie points, so I said, 'Yes, I've learned a great deal today. Staff Nurse explains things well.'

'Dr Wolfbane told me about the paper underpants incident.'

Feeling my face transform into a flaming mask, I half choked on my next words. 'I'm . . . I'm sorry I didn't help Mr Harefield dress for theatre. I don't know where he got the paper pants.'

'Something to tell the grandchildren, I think?' she said, with a glimmer of a smile.

I nodded meekly. 'Yes, Sister.'

'And be careful of Wolfbane. He was asking about you. He can be . . . obsessive with young nurses. You might want to lose the blusher and mascara for tomorrow.'

'Yes, Sister,' I said, staring at my feet.

'Off you go, Johnson,' she ordered.

'Thank you, Sister,' I said, and skedaddled.

Before leaving, I went to see Gavin. He was looking sorry for himself. There were two bands of tape across a white dressing on his nose.

'Can I get you anything?' I asked.

'A new head would be good.'

'Did you do the paper underpants thing as a joke?' I asked, smiling so he would know I wasn't cross.

'Not really,' he said. 'There wasn't a paper theatre hat with the gown you gave me so I used a pair of paper pants. My mother gave me a bag of them to use while I'm in hospital. Did I get you into trouble?'

'No, gosh, no, Gavin,' I said. 'It was pretty funny.'

He tried to smile, but it hurt.

Outside the rain had stopped, but the cold wind hadn't and it was already dark when I walked down to Camberwell Green. A steady stream of buses and cars whooshed past me, their headlights beaming a yellowish glow on the wet road. I stopped at a Wimpy bar and bought Tilly a strawberry milkshake, then continued on home, dodging puddles and splashes from the road.

I couldn't wait to see how Adele, Miranda and Kathy had fared on their first day at St Francis. I knew

Jan would have had no problems at Dulwich. Her irrepressible good humour would have charmed even the most officious ward sister. At St Giles, Polly would have quietly got on with everything she was told to do, Laurel would have given at least two people what-for in her inimitable cheeky manner, and Meredith would have learned more than any of us.

I was thinking that life was particularly good. I had done a good day's work, had good friends I couldn't wait to see, and a boyfriend I couldn't wait to hold. Out of nowhere, a wave of unbridled pleasure swept over me.

CHAPTER 7

The Long Slow March
of Feminism

King's College Hospital, London: Early 1971

ON THE EVENING of our first day on our new wards, my
friends and I met at our usual haunt, the Fox on the
Hill, to compare notes.

Warm and cosy, the pub was nevertheless unwel-
coming to us. Women in pubs without male company
were viewed with suspicion and, apart from the bar-
maid, we were the only females in the lounge. The
subject of intense scrutiny from fellow drinkers, we
knew the landlord could refuse to serve us, which was
why we hadn't dared invade the testosterone-dripping
public bar, where working-class men shared pints with
their mates.

'Make way for the Babycham Brigade,' remarked a
thirty-something man in a suit. His friends standing
with him at the bar laughed and eyed us up for possible
availability. For sure, they had already sprayed
everything in the room with their scent.

Ignoring the unwanted attention, we settled at a

table near the window with our half-pints of lager and packets of crisps. The landlord wouldn't serve us pints.

'It's absolutely awful at Franny's,' Miranda complained about St Francis. Miranda, like Polly, was training to be a health visitor, a qualification that tacked an extra year on to their training.

I felt sad for my friends. Adele, Miranda and Kathy were not impressed with their geriatric wards at St Francis, and Polly, Laurel, Meredith, Jan and I made sympathetic noises as they described the heavy work I knew so well from Dickens.

'It was much worse than I anticipated,' Adele said. She stood up to look out of the window for any sign of Fraser's car. Adele wanted to be a midwife, which would add another two years to her training. That was five years of hiding a husband, for which, if she achieved it, I thought she should be awarded an OBE. 'I've never worked so damn hard in my life,' she whined, as she sat back down.

'I feel sorry for the old people living at Franny's,' Kathy said. 'At least we get to leave at the end of the day.'

'I wish men would stop staring at us,' Meredith interjected. She looked pointedly at the bald gentleman at the next table, who was nursing a pint and watching us closely.

'Poop, shit, crap, fart, tit, bum,' Laurel said loudly, and the bald man quickly looked away. 'That worked,' she said. She took off her glasses and wiped them with a hanky that she then stuffed dramatically into her bra.

'Well, I had a good day,' Jan said, to brighten things up a bit. 'My ward at Dulwich was great and I learned a lot.'

'Like what?' Meredith asked, keeping the positive conversation going.

'Like I'm going out to dinner tomorrow night.'

'Who with?' Kathy asked. She took a dainty sip of beer and looked relieved the subject had changed.

'Yes, who with?' Miranda wanted to know.

'What is this? Twenty Questions?' Jan remarked, feigning indignation.

'I don't want to know,' Adele said petulantly, and stood up again to look for Fraser. They were having dinner with friends in Lewisham.

'Yes, you do,' Jan teased, 'and sit down. You're like a bloody yo-yo.'

'Okay, I do want to know,' Adele admitted, and sat down again.

'Me too,' Meredith said.

Polly, I noticed, was very quiet, lost in her own world over something.

'So, are you going to tell us his name?' I asked Jan.

'Uh-huh.' She grinned broadly at me. 'His name's Digby, and he's a doctor.'

'Digby!' we all screeched. 'Digby!'

We pulled Jan's leg over his name and extracted every detail of his invitation.

'Mr Nosy Baldy Parker at the next table is listening to everything we're saying,' Miranda reminded us. Sometimes we could be quite ribald on half a pint.

'I think we should arm-wrestle,' Meredith said. 'Really give him something to take home.'

'Can anyone be bothered?' Laurel asked.

Collectively deciding against a show of strength, we finished the Digby subject, and I told them about Gavin and the paper pants fiasco, leaving out my concerns about Wolfbane. Laurel and Adele laughed so hard I thought they were going to lay eggs.

'Why don't women have paper bras and pants to protect their dignity in the operating theatre?' Kathy asked out of the blue.

We all looked at her. It was, perhaps, one of the most relevant and telling questions ever asked about female patients.

'I don't think anyone has thought of it,' Meredith said.

'Because men are in charge and women's modesty doesn't matter?' Laurel suggested.

Kathy nodded sagely. 'We have a long way to go, ladies.'

'We certainly do,' I said, thinking I should probably write and tell Germaine Greer about this.

'If men had periods,' Laurel said, 'there would be a contest to see who had the heaviest flow.'

In agreement, I quipped, 'And they'd award a medal to the winner.'

Our jesting was interrupted by the arrival of Kip and his friends Danny and Roman, both university students whom we all already knew.

'There's a nurses' party in Herne Hill later,' Danny announced, as he placed a tray of beers on the table, pints for the boys, halves for us. Tall and fit-looking, with fashionably long brown hair and a Liverpool accent, he pulled out a chair and sat down next to Miranda. Kip and Roman dragged two empty chairs from another table, and Meredith and I made space for them.

'We can have supper at the King's refectory, then get a bus to Herne Hill,' Danny said, taking charge of our social engagements. Danny loved the hospital food, which amused us no end. It was his idea of going out to dinner.

'We can't arrive at the party before eleven,' Kathy reminded us.

'No way,' Jan agreed. Arriving too early could seriously damage our groovy image.

Adele stood up again. 'Here's Fraser,' she said and struggled into her Afghan coat. 'See ya. Have a fun night,' she added, as she hurried away. There was a blast of cold air as the door opened.

Polly hadn't touched her beer. I was about to ask her what was wrong when Kathy said, 'I wonder why female nurses aren't allowed to catheterize male patients?' Discrimination was obviously playing on her mind.

Roman almost choked on his beer and I grinned at him. An olive-skinned, dark-haired lad of Ukrainian heritage, he was probably the smartest of us all. Quiet, well-mannered and shy, he seemed unnerved by Kathy's question.

'Well?' Kathy demanded, when no one had responded. She was an expert at provoking thought and making us question our opinions and ideals. If she hadn't been so good at sewing, I would have told her to take up confrontational ethics as a hobby.

'It's because blokes wouldn't like it,' Danny ventured, and Kip nodded.

'Well, I don't particularly like the idea of a man looking at my fundaments either,' Miranda said.

'But that's different,' Kip argued.

'No, it's not. Kathy has a point,' Laurel said, being serious for once. 'If male doctors can catheterize both men and women, why can't female nurses do both as well?'

We women knew what the men were thinking:

that the mechanics of their marvellous manhood were far too complex for a female to understand. The ancient patriarchal wheels were going round in their heads, but none of them was brave enough to voice his true thoughts.

'Darts?' Jan asked eventually, looking around hopefully.

'I'm in,' I said, and stood up.

As we collected the darts, the low rumble of blokey banter in the background stopped and the group of middle-aged banker-types at the bar gawped at us. Unfazed, Jan started to elaborately exercise her arms as though she were about to perform on parallel bars. 'I must, I must, increase my bust,' she chanted loudly, as she pumped her arms.

Laughing, I said, 'Do you think they're wondering if we can throw over-arm?'

'Nah,' Jan said, stopping to wipe the scoreboard. 'They're worried the banks will soon allow us to take out a mortgage on our own.'

'If you play badly, Maggie,' Kip called out, 'you could probably wing one of those suits at the bar from there.'

Pleased by his support, and aware I was playing to a full house, I threw my first dart and tried not to watch Jan, who was now touching her toes. I hit as close to the bullseye as I was ever going to get, and I felt the rewarding rush of satisfaction that comes with success that has been witnessed by those who would wish otherwise. Of course, my next two shots hit the board and dropped to the floor, but you can't have everything.

Shortly, the others joined us at the dartboard and

we rotated teams until hunger pains drove us to walk over to the refectory at King's.

I caught up with Polly as we crossed Denmark Hill. 'What's up?' I asked her.

'Is it obvious?'

'Uh-huh.'

'I've finished with James,' she said, the words catching in her throat. 'But I wish I hadn't.'

A verbal response from me was unnecessary. I linked arms with Polly as we walked. Over the coming years, we would all be falling in and out of love. Some relationships would hurt. Some would be fleeting and leave no mark. Some would endure.

And if they didn't, and we had wanted them to, there would always be one of us there to pick up the pieces.

Such was life in those first six months in London.

Not long after I started on Fisk and Cheere, I developed swollen neck glands, a high fever and an inflamed sore throat. This was unusual, as I was a robust human and couldn't recall ever having had a cold. Following Sister Marybeth's dire warning about throat infections on the ward, I reported to sick bay at King's.

Throat swabs and bloods were taken, glandular fever was diagnosed, and I was packed off home. Jan put me on the train at Waterloo and my mother met me at Fareham station with a blanket, a hot-water bottle and a packet of aspirin. She had just returned from visiting my father in Rotterdam and was keen to have her wayward child trapped in bed, where she could talk me out of going back to nursing.

'I'll think about it,' I said, as Mum delivered hot chocolate and strawberry ice cream to my sick bed.

'You're probably right,' I agreed, as rhubarb crumble and lashings of custard were placed in front of me.

'I'm considering going back to school and finishing my A levels,' I mused aloud, as crème caramel, lemon mousse, and bread and butter pudding appeared on a tray.

'I'm going back to London,' I said ten days later when I felt a bit better.

After that, it was canned tomato soup with a tablespoon.

I'd been back at work a week when Gavin Harefield walked on to the ward with a box of chocolates for the nurses. Gavin was a great-looking guy now that his nose was fixed and, emboldened by his new leading-man looks, he asked our gorgeous Staff Nurse Carter out. Dating patients, even after discharge, was a no-no, and Julia (who was already taken) turned poor Gavin down. It does make you wonder how nurses married their patients during the war, doesn't it? Perhaps dating rules were suspended for the duration.

As I feared, the cadaverous Dr Wolfbane pursued me even after I had twice refused a date. If he wasn't pestering me when I took a patient to theatre, he arrived on the ward and stood by the file trolley, pretending to look at notes. When I walked past, he would reach out and touch my arm under the pretence of needing to ask a question. Regardless of whether it was a genuine enquiry, I consistently ignored him and kept going. I had to. As a paper cap I would have been keel-hauled by a sister if I was by myself and seen talking to a doctor on the ward. Considered ignorant of all information, I wasn't even allowed to answer the telephone.

One miserably chilly afternoon when I was walking home to St Giles, Wolfbane pulled over in his car and offered me a lift. The cold made his offer tempting, but good sense prevailed and I refused, rather rudely: 'You'd need to wear a tablecloth to get laid, you loathsome creep,' I said, with quiet savagery. Okay, I didn't say that. What I said was, 'Go away, please,' but I wish I'd said the other thing.

In a strange way, he was making me feel guilty, as if I were somehow at fault, and because of this I refrained from mentioning the problem to Kip and my friends in case they thought I was conceited and encouraging him.

Brad Hutchins, the male staff nurse on Fisk, became aware of my Wolfbane problem one early duty. Brad was sitting at the nurses' desk and I was standing next to him when Wolfbane stopped opposite us. Brad looked up and saw Wolfbane staring at the name badge pinned to my apron over my right breast.

'Hmm, Nurse Johnson,' Wolfbane said, with a lewd intonation. 'What do you call the other one?'

'Hey!' Brad said sharply.

Not the least bothered, Wolfbane laughed and walked away.

'Does he need sorting?' Brad asked me.

I had no doubt that Brad could fell a charging bull, but I declined his offer because whenever anyone got 'sorted' on Z Cars, they ended up in traction. As a mature woman – or at least a young woman who was growing up quickly – I believed I could deal with Wolfbane's unwanted attentions on my own. Famous last words.

'That bugger reminds me of someone,' Brad mused.

'Me too,' I said.

Unexpectedly, the romance between Julia and Dr Brown came to an abrupt end. Heartbroken, within a week Julia transferred to the Belgrave Hospital for Children, and a month later moved to Scotland.

After her departure, Brad picked up my education on the nursing front, and between us we went overboard with practising procedures. Supervised by him, I removed stitches and staples, and mastered the intricate dismantling of the long, continual stitch that some surgeons preferred. I assisted him with sterile dressings on heads, necks, ears and noses, removed drains from wounds, gave injections, syringed ears, shaved men prior to surgery, took countless patients to theatre and looked after them when they returned to the ward. I acted as second-fiddle on drug rounds, assisted at a cardiac arrest (I noted what drugs were administered), wrote in the Kardex and pushed suppositories (or 'sweeties for bum-bums', as Brad called them) into a variety of bottoms. I only ever cleaned equipment on afternoons when the ward was quiet, and I never did it alone.

'Did Fenella receive a good ward report?' I asked Brad, while we were removing staples from a thyroid-ectomy wound on my last day. I knew Sister Marybeth had consulted him before writing my report, and that he was responsible for her encouraging words.

'Of course,' Brad said, 'and it was much, much better than yours.'

'You are a beast,' I said, grinning at him. But I knew it would have been. Fenella was a born nurse.

As my time on Fisk and Cheere came to an end, so

did my relationship with Kip. He was a fabulous, thoughtful, handsome man – all the good things – but I was scared of any intense romance that might influence the future I had chosen. I wanted a career, and to dictate my own path in life and make choices based on my own needs. It was still very much a man's world, and time and again I had met women who had abandoned their dreams to further those of a man.

Selfish? Sensible? Womens' rights gone mad?

All three, perhaps. But what if I suddenly decided to spend a year in Alaska training sled dogs for the Iditarod? Would a boyfriend drop his degree to work in a bar in Anchorage to support me?

Exactly!

CHAPTER 8

Pantia Ralli, Pantia Ralli

Ibiza and London: Spring and Summer 1971

'I'M GLAD THAT exam's over,' I told Miranda, as we joined the throng of students spilling out of the School of Nursing at the end of our first training block since PTS. 'What the hell is an abdominal insertion anyway?'

'It was a typing mistake,' she said, laughing. 'It should have been abdominal incision.'

'Oh, bugger. I thought it was a wound drain.'

Unlike final state exams, which were administered externally, our block exams were set and marked by our tutors. Only eight months into our training, there was much at stake as we had to pass every exam to continue.

'I can't wait to get out of here,' Jan said, joining us. 'I'm stuffed!'

'Me too,' I said. Exhausted from hard work on the wards, lack of sleep after all-night parties, and weeks of lectures and study in block, we were all ready for a break. Kathy and I had found a reasonably priced package tour to Ibiza in the Balearic Islands, where the sea was warm, the wine was cold and the sun shone every day. It was exactly what we needed.

Of my other friends, some were staying in London and some were travelling. Not one of us was prepared for Laurel's travel plan – especially me, and I should have seen it coming . . .

Laurel and I had become good buddies since those fledgling days of PTS, and she sometimes travelled home with me to Fareham. She enjoyed my mother's company and, being a homebody, I think that from time to time Laurel needed the warmth and security of a real family home around her.

My mother, in turn, adored Laurel, an affection evidenced by the frenzy of 'cookie' catering that preceded Laurel's arrival and the best Irish linen sheets that were put on Laurel's bed. One time, we even had hot dogs and my mother bought a bottle of tomato ketchup. It was the talk of Fareham.

My father was mostly away at sea on those visits home, and Mum's cousin, my aunt Joan, would occasionally make up a female foursome at dinner. It was hysterical listening to my mother, aunt and friend batting funny stories back and forth across the table. We laughed well into the night, and none of it was repeatable.

Then one morning my mother found Laurel weeping in bed. Inconsolable, Laurel told us she was missing her family and boyfriend in Canada. At length, Mum and I talked her into staying and finishing her training, but in the end homesickness and love proved too big a burden, and Laurel flew home on the day Kathy and I flew to Ibiza.

Laurel was one of the wittiest girls I had ever met and her sudden departure left a huge void in all our lives.

It was the following spring when my mother finally threw away the bottle of tomato ketchup.

Salty-skinned and sleepy, I closed *Papillon*, the book I was reading, lay on my side and watched the middle-aged couple who were chatting next to me – a large British woman in a crochet bikini and a man wearing Union Jack swimming trunks. Was there anybody left in England? As far as the eye could see, the beach at Santa Eulalia del Río was littered with holidaying Brits.

'Do you want to swim out to the raft?' Kathy asked.

'Maybe.' I sighed and rolled on to my back.

Wearing bikinis, the two of us were lying side by side, marinating in coconut oil and roasting like sausages on a grill. I stared up at the cloudless sky, hoping the nothingness would settle the jumble of thoughts in my head. I was upset about Laurel. I was concerned that I might have failed the block exam. And I couldn't stop thinking about Kip. I was missing him something awful.

Shielding my eyes from the sun, I sat up and looked at the raft tethered a hundred yards offshore. Deserted, it looked tempting, bobbing about on the water. 'Race you,' I challenged Kathy.

Scrambling to our feet, we ran down the beach and threw ourselves into the water. Neck and neck most of the way, we climbed the ladder and lay on the raft like spent seals, laughing and panting in the bright sunlight.

The swim out to the raft was to become a daily adventure to our own little island in paradise. On land, we avoided the masses by exploring the backstreets of the old town, cycling across fields to swim at secluded beaches, and lunching at local cafés on gazpacho, paella and garlic squid, which we washed down with fruity sangria.

All too soon, it was time to return to London. As the plane rose over the island, I gazed down at the ragged coastline and the blue-water wonderland. Goodbye, sunshine . . .

Hello, St Giles nurses' home on fire!

Fortunately no one was hurt, but the smoke damage was extensive and many of us were to be moved to another nurses' home. No explanation was provided about how the fire had started, but gossip was that the culprit was a patient whose advances had been spurned by a nurse.

Which nurse? we wanted to know. We knew everyone's business and it wasn't anyone we'd heard about. Over the moon that all of us had passed the block exam, I stopped caring about the identity of the spurning nurse and started wondering whether we might be allowed to move out of the nurses' home instead of relocating.

Fat chance! We were speedily rehoused, along with Sister Morag, in the nurses' home on the top floor above the main entrance at King's. And a lovely surprise awaited me. Jan moved from Dulwich into the room next to mine, Kathy and Adele (plus Fraser) were in rooms further along the corridor, Tilly was opposite me, and Meredith was next to her. Unfortunately, Miranda and Polly were still at St Giles as their rooms hadn't been damaged.

Our new rooms were large and modern with psychedelic wallpaper, new washbasins, fitted carpet and decent furnishings. They had been upgraded for senior unmarried staff, many of whom, like Sister Morag, had lived in for most of their lives. As there was nowhere else to put us, we had struck lucky.

Or had we?

Two weeks later, we were woken at 2 a.m. by the fire alarm. Someone had set fire to clothes in the laundry on our corridor. My jeans were a goner. Rushing downstairs to the evacuation point in the main nurses' sitting room, we stood tall in our dressing-gowns while Fraser hid behind us in his pyjamas. Luckily Sister Morag was at her sister's in Scotland. Luckily – because three male medical students also appeared. Naturally we were all totally shocked – even the nurses whose beds they had been in.

The fire was quickly extinguished and we returned to our rooms. Nothing was said about the men as it was assumed they had come from the rooms where on-call doctors stayed – rooms that could be reached by back stairs at one end of our corridor. How daft was that?

Over the next few weeks, there were two more fires and a nurse from my set was attacked during the night as she returned to her room from the bathroom. She was found unconscious on the floor behind her bedroom door, her nightdress ripped and razor cuts carved on her upper back.

Again, the rumour was of a spurned gentleman. Then the story changed to a vengeful man whose wife had died at King's. Then it was a satanic lunatic. Petrified, we started sleeping two and three to a room. With hockey sticks. And more medical students.

The nurse who was attacked transferred her training to another hospital, and I never heard of her again. To my knowledge, the culprit was never caught, but the fires stopped, there were no further attacks and slowly everything returned to normal.

Not long after the fires, I went to a party in Tulse Hill with friends. Kip was there and our eyes met across a crowded room. Smiling, he made his way towards me and my spirits lifted. But as he moved closer his smile rapidly faded and turned into an anxious frown. 'Oh, I'm terribly sorry,' Kip said. 'I thought you were some-one else.'

'Who?' I demanded crossly. I could feel tears welling up.

'My great aunt Mildred,' he said.

Kip managed about five seconds before the corners of his mouth started to quiver with laughter and he whisked me on to the dance floor.

Ain't love grand!

That summer, I was sent to Pantia Ralli, a female surgi-cal ward at King's. It was a large old Nightingale ward, and the most enjoyable part of working on Pantia Ralli was the wonderful name. At home, at the shops and in restaurants, I couldn't say 'Pantia Ralli' enough.

There was a high patient turnover and a broad range of surgical nursing to learn: heart, bowel, lungs, pancreas, stomach, spleen and gall bladder, to name a few body parts. There was also cardiothoracic surgery, and I was so proud of nursing a patient who had received a mitral valve replacement that I, the obvious heroine of the piece, wrote about it in excruciating detail to my mother.

The major downside to cardiac operations was

that patients had most of their teeth removed prior to surgery, but this wasn't as alarming as it sounds. Owing to poor diet and dental care during and after the Second World War, many middle-aged and older patients already had false teeth, and any remaining teeth that had decayed were removed to prevent dangerous infection attacking the heart.

As a general rule, if you lived in Camberwell and were female, fair, fat, forty and fertile, at some point you would be admitted to Pantia Ralli to have your gall bladder whipped out. It was a nasty little organ that filled with stones and caused no end of pain and sickness. Post-operative recovery was slow and uncomfortable, with tubes and drains and a good-sized wound.

Finally having escaped the shadow of my colleague – the capable and diligent Fenella – within a week of starting on Pantia Ralli I was changing surgical dressings, giving enemas and passing flatus tubes into blocked and windy bottoms, assisting senior nurses to insert catheters into bladders and naso-gastric tubes into stomachs, and answering the ward phone. Nurse Johnson speaking. Oh yeah!

I also witnessed my first operation while working on Pantia Ralli – a splenectomy (removal of spleen) – and the operating theatre was a revelation. I had expected a tense, dramatic atmosphere with blood squirting everywhere and impatient surgeons demanding instruments from frazzled nurses. But I was wrong. The theatre was relaxed, Cat Stevens playing in the background and cheerful banter among the staff.

What I hadn't expected was blasted Dr Wolfbane at the top end of the operating table. Our eyes met over our masks. Mine narrowed. I still couldn't figure out who he reminded me of.

As soon as Wolfbane knew I was on Pantia Ralli, he became a nuisance again. Nicknamed Dr Wolfman by one of the patients, Wolfbane started passing me notes on the ward – notes that I promptly binned. He also began appearing as I was going off duty. This posed a real problem, as I didn't want him to know I lived at King's. As a foil, and even though it was summer, I performed an elaborate charade, putting on my nurse's coat and beret as I left the ward. Then, looking like Scott of the Antarctic, I walked out of the hospital main entrance, ran along to the nurses'-home door, disappeared inside and took the lift to my room.

On the ward, Wolfbane's attentions had not gone unnoticed, and one morning Sister Caroline called me to her office. I had no idea what I had done wrong.

'Nurse Johnson,' she said, her manner helpful rather than cross. 'I think you should be aware that your boyfriend Dr Wolfbane is married. And he should not be visiting you on the ward.'

I was stunned. Ugh! They thought Wolfbane was my boyfriend!

Taking a seat, I related my tale of woe. From the way Sister Caroline was nodding, I gathered she had heard a similar story before.

'Leave it with me,' Sister Caroline said confidently, and whatever she did or said worked because the creep stopped bothering me – for almost a year.

Wolfbane aside, I enjoyed my time on Pantia Ralli. I was even toying with the idea that surgical nursing might be my forte. The work was interesting and rewarding without being too physically demanding – mostly, though, I just wanted to say I worked on a ward called Pantia Ralli.

With summer in full swing, there was fun to be had in London. Kip and I poshed up for a summer ball; Jan, Polly and I went to watch tennis at Wimbledon; and Miranda, Danny, Kip and I went rowing on the Serpentine. My parents had recently moved to a house in Hindhead, Surrey, and Jan, Polly and I hitched down to visit them a few times – most of our lifts were from elderly women and country vicars driving Morris Minors who were worried about us hitching.

It was quite the thing in fashion terms to buy hipster jeans that were too small, lie on the floor to struggle into them, pull the zipper up with a coat-hanger, climb into the bath to wet the jeans, then climb out and let the jeans mould to your body as they dried. It was the most effective contraceptive ever devised, and, once dressed, you couldn't sit down or go to the loo.

Rumours abounded that tight jeans could make men infertile and cause vaginal thrush in women, but we took no notice. Who knew that the hip pain, numbness and tingling in our thighs that some of us felt was compression of the femoral cutaneous nerve in our hips, a direct result of wearing tight hipster jeans? It became known as tight-pants syndrome.

The discomfort didn't stop Jan, Kathy and me wearing our super-tight jeans to the free Grand Funk Railroad, Humble Pie and Heads Hands & Feet concert in Hyde Park. It rained so hard that we couldn't sit down anyway, and it was safer to be standing when Hell's Angels started throwing cans and bottles. Peter

Frampton and Humble Pie were worth the tube fare and an exploding bladder.

It was also about this time I received a letter from Lloyds bank advising that I was overdrawn by £18.60. I nearly died. How could this be? Oh, the disgrace . . .

Frantic, and already picturing myself sleeping in a cardboard box at Waterloo station, I called the Duchess of Milton Keynes (or whoever my mother was that week). After insisting I should be more careful with money, she advised me to see the bank manager to arrange repayment.

A bank manager? I couldn't possibly talk to a *bank manager*!

So I talked to the teller, who talked to the bank manager, who took my weeping personage to his office. A bank manager's office. I nearly fainted. And he looked like Boris Karloff with a crew cut, which didn't help.

Several cheques printed with my name, which I had signed, were handed to me. I fumbled through the pile and stopped at a cheque made out for £20 cash. The signature on it wasn't even in my name.

'This is not mine,' I said, passing the cheque to Boris. 'It's signed by someone called Bernard Ballon!'

'No, it isn't your signature,' he agreed. 'You had better inform the police.'

Me?

My meekness was quickly replaced with disgust at the manager's lack of responsibility and assistance. Furious, I went straight to Scotland Yard.

'Has the bank refunded your money?' Detective Mike Rogers asked me. His daughter was a nurse at Guy's.

I shook my head. 'Do they have to?'

He nodded. 'You'd better leave this with me.'

Leaving my problems with other people was really working for me, and a week later the missing funds were returned to my account.

Detective Rogers advised me that Bernard Ballon, another nurse's boyfriend, had entered my room while I was in the bath, opened the staples in my chequebook, removed the last cheque and carefully re-closed the staples. He had then cashed the stolen cheque at my bank in Camberwell.

'The teller should have noticed that you'd suddenly turned into a man called Bernard,' Mike Rogers told me.

Oh, how we laughed.

It was apparent from the start of my training that I was never going to be the poster girl for British nursing, but despite glandular fever, a bad ward report from Dickens, and my challenge to the archaic system of using student nurses as cheap cleaning labour, I'd survived the first year.

For this achievement, I was rewarded with a frilly hat to signify my status as a second-year student nurse. Designed by a blind milliner, the white linen confection came with a wad of blue tissue stuffing to keep it high and proud. From a distance, I looked like I was wearing a wedding cake on my head, but I didn't care. If I had to wear silly hats to finish my training, so be it: I loved nursing and I was going to qualify come Hell or high water. I can't recall a precise moment when I realized how much the job meant to me; it was more a slow revelation that seemed to happen without me even being aware of it.

CHAPTER 9

The Elephant in the Womb

Dulwich Hospital, London: October 1971

I HAD PASSED my intermediate exams, and another chilly autumn was taking hold when I walked into Dulwich Hospital to begin my gynaecology training. I knew the hospital well from the School of Nursing, and I skipped up the stairs like a local.

Like Pantia Ralli at King's, the gynae ward at Dulwich had a high patient turnover, and morning report promised a busy day. Patients with uterine prolapse (the uterus had collapsed into the vagina), fibroids (benign uterine tumours), ovarian cysts, endometriosis (the uterine lining was growing outside the uterus) and incomplete miscarriage (where tissue was retained) were listed for surgery, and others with heavy bleeding, abdominal pain and infertility were earmarked for investigations. In our last block, we had covered the female reproductive system and I had learned about the associated diseases and treatments available, so I had an idea what to expect.

Or so I thought.

'Close the door and sit down, Johnson,' Sister Sonya ordered, as I turned to leave the office after report. Her unfriendly face was heavily made-up, and there was an air of stand-offish superiority about her that was disturbing. I guessed she was in her mid-thirties.

I sat down and smoothed my crisp white apron.

'Are you a Catholic?' she demanded.

'Why do you ask, Sister?'

'Don't answer a question with a question,' she said crossly.

'No, I'm not Catholic.' I was instantly wary.

'Do you have any objection to assisting with pregnancy terminations?'

Ah, so that was it. The Abortion Act had been passed in 1967, legalizing abortion and thereby saving the lives of countless women who would have sought the assistance of backstreet abortionists. The graveyards of London were littered with the bodies of desperate women who had contracted sepsis and died slowly in terrible pain, or bled to death, too scared to seek help and admit to what was then a crime.

Abortion hadn't been mentioned in class, although it might have been taught the day I skived off and went to an exhibition at the Hayward Gallery with my mother. Consequently I was unprepared for this sudden interrogation. I had no idea what sort of nursing was involved in a termination, and no notion of my own opinions, as I had not had time to develop any.

However, having had Rosie O'Brien bend my ear on Dickens over the sin of judgement, I refused to allow personal sensitivities to affect my training or patient care. I wasn't looking forward to seeing an aborted foetus – who would? – but I wasn't eager to witness an eye operation either. I had always been squeamish about eyes.

'No, no problem, Sister,' I said. Intrigued, I asked, 'But what if I did have objections?'

'The only permitted training exclusion is Catholicism,' Sister Sonya said flatly.

'That's unfair,' I countered, before I could stop myself.

Shut up, Maggie. Shut up, shut up, SHUT UP!

A frown formed on Sister's brow. 'I agree,' she said, surprising me. 'The ruling only considers the nurse. It wouldn't be fair on a patient to have a hostile nurse regardless of religion, so if you didn't want to be involved—'

'You wouldn't make me,' I finished for her.

'No!' she said sharply. 'I wouldn't *allow* you to be involved. And don't interrupt again. Now go to work!'

With food for thought, I walked on to the busy ward and looked around. A typical Nightingale set-up, the patients' beds were positioned around the perimeter of the ward, with curtains that could be pulled around each bed. Physical privacy was difficult and verbal privacy impossible. Everyone knew everyone else's bodily secrets, especially after a doctor's round.

With several patients to prepare for theatre and six from the day before to monitor, bath and ambulate, there were nurses criss-crossing the ward like they were doing a country dance.

One of the magical things nursing was teaching me, and I wasn't even conscious of it, was the ability to walk on to a ward and see at a glance what needed to be done. Spotting a kipper making a bed alone, I went to assist. Her name, she told me, was Eleanor. 'I can't be doing with last names,' she said.

I smiled. 'Me neither. I'm not in the army.'

She smiled back. The frilly and the kipper were going to get along fine.

In her late twenties, Eleanor was older than most third-year students and had worked as an air hostess before switching to nursing. This explained her confident air, the perfectly groomed short blonde hair and the luminous skin. Unfortunately the perennial tools of nursing, soap and water, had done a number on her hands.

Working in tandem, we examined wound dressings for leakage, checked sanitary pads and estimated blood loss, removed alternate sutures on a seven-day post-op patient, and prepared two women for abdominal hysterectomies.

Men usually had only a watch and a wallet to lock away while they were in theatre, but women possessed numerous items of jewellery that needed to be listed and secured in the DDA cupboard, where dangerous drugs were kept (DDA standing for Dangerous Drugs Act).

'Always write *yellow* metal ring, never gold,' Eleanor told me. 'In case anyone says they've been given back a fake.'

'Good grief. Who would do that?' I said.

'This is South London,' Eleanor replied, as though it was the fraud capital of the known world.

While Eleanor took Mrs Wagstaff to theatre for removal of an ovarian cyst, I shaved a very hairy, middle-aged, no-nonsense Londoner called Mrs Barnes from her nipples to her knees prior to hysterectomy.

'Dear me,' Mrs Barnes said, when I was shaving between her legs. 'Is it really necessary to mow the lady garden?'

Hiding a grin, I said, 'The surgeon has requested it.'

Shaving wasn't easy, particularly the difficult terrain on a woman's body where there are more hills and valleys than the Himalayas. Terrified of cutting Mrs Barnes, I took far too much time, but I did learn that my patient was known for her apricot dainties and prize-winning dahlias.

'As long as you did it properly,' Eleanor reassured me, when she returned from theatre.

'And as long as they take this blasted utensil out of me,' Mrs Barnes said anxiously, as she struggled into the theatre gown. 'Our Carol's getting hitched next Saturday and I've got to make apricot dainties.'

'It's called a uterus, Mrs Barnes,' Eleanor said helpfully.

I pulled the theatre cap over our patient's head and tucked in stray blue curls. Both Eleanor and I were aware that it was in the lap of the gods whether Mrs Barnes would be at her daughter's wedding or not. Even after a blood transfusion, she was still ghostly pale, although her blood count was good enough for surgery to proceed. More blood was cross-matched and prepared in case she needed it.

For over a month, Mrs Barnes had experienced heavy menstrual bleeding and severe pain. Busy with preparations for the family wedding, she had done nothing about the problem except put wads of old hand-towels between her legs and take painkillers. Finally collapsing from loss of blood, she was admitted to hospital, where a large uterine mass was detected.

The Elephant in the Womb

Mrs Barnes was warned that the surgeon might also remove her ovaries, and to prepare herself that the mass might be cancerous.

'When am I going to theatre?' Mrs Barnes asked.

'Mrs Wagstaff is first on the list,' Eleanor said, opening the curtains, 'and you're third, so in about an hour.'

'Is Mrs Wagstaff the lady with the Bavarian cyst?'

'That's her,' Eleanor said, with a giggle.

Our other hysterectomy patient was Debra Cadogan. Twenty-two, unmarried and a physical education teacher, Debra had endometriosis that was causing disabling pain and excessive menstrual bleeding. Her illness was curtailing her sporting activities, making her life a living hell.

Removal of her uterus would resolve the endometriosis but also render her incapable of having a child. There was no counselling available if Debra had concerns about this, which she obviously did.

'I can always adopt,' she said gaily when, overseen by Eleanor, I gave her the pre-med injection. 'Anyway, I don't like children.'

Eleanor flashed me a look. I didn't know what to say.

'It doesn't worry me,' Debra went on nervously. 'Even if the nursery is gone, the playpen will still be open.'

I gave a cursory laugh at her joke. Eleanor didn't react at all. I couldn't begin to imagine what I would do in the same situation. At that time, there was no such thing as harvesting eggs and freezing them for future *in vitro* fertilization and possible surrogacy.

'Have you had a second opinion?' Eleanor asked her.

Debra nodded. 'Three opinions with the same

recommendation: hysterectomy. Just think, I won't have to worry about periods.'

'That's good news,' I said, and smiled. I had no idea how to support Debra through this. Platitudes didn't remotely cut the mustard.

While Eleanor removed stitches and a wound drain, I removed two indwelling urinary catheters. When the women had both passed urine, I went to find Sister and report it. She was serving tea from a feeder cup to a woman dying of ovarian cancer. The patient was lying on her side, propped up with pillows. Only fifty, Merrivale Field was emaciated and subdued by Brompton's cocktail, a mixture that included heroin, cocaine and gin to control pain in the terminally ill. I smiled at Mrs Field but there was no response. Her eyes were sunken and there were tufts of brown hair on her scalp. How awful, I thought, to die so publicly.

'Would you like me to take over, Sister?' I asked.

'No, thank you, Johnson,' she said softly. 'I'm telling Merrivale about my camellias. We both like camellias.'

Gosh. Might Sister Sonya be a softy inside?

Suddenly a young woman cried out in pain and every available nurse on the ward headed for her bed. Eleanor and I arrived first.

Pulling the curtains, Eleanor said, 'Fetch a bedpan, Maggie, quickly!'

Walking fast, I grabbed a pan and paper cover and returned to the bedside.

Nineteen-year-old Sally had received medication the previous afternoon that would, within twenty-four hours, dilate her cervix and expel the foetus she was carrying. Her contractions to abort had just started.

The Elephant in the Womb

There was an IV infusion in her arm, so Eleanor and I helped her on to the bedpan.

'Couldn't we slot the pan into a commode so Sally is more comfortable?' I asked Eleanor.

'No, she needs to be on the bed in case of problems.'

There were already problems, I thought. What about the fact that everyone could hear Sally's private experience? What about the poor woman in the next bed who was having investigations for infertility? What must she be thinking?

Another kipper came in with a stack of large sanitary pads and put them on the bedside locker. She smiled kindly at Sally. 'Need anything else?' she asked Eleanor.

'Can you take the woman in the next bed for a walk along the corridor?' Eleanor asked.

'No need. Staff has already taken her and the incomplete miscarriage to the day room.'

Nurses often referred to patients by their diagnosis. The incomplete miscarriage had occurred at six months' gestation. A dilation and curettage (D and C) was performed to remove remaining tissue from her uterus.

'Thank God,' Sally said. 'I couldn't bear to have them witness this.' Seized by a strong contraction, she cried out in pain.

I stayed with Sally while Eleanor took another patient to theatre. I was terrified. So was Sally. Drenched in sweat and gripping my hand, she tried to muffle her cries while I said helpful things like 'There, there' and 'You'll be fine'. Next block, I was going to ask for some role play to cover situations like this.

Eleanor rejoined us a few minutes before the foetus was expelled into the bedpan.

'Don't look,' Eleanor told Sally. She quickly covered the bedpan with the paper cover and disappeared outside the curtains.

I placed a pad between Sally's legs and pulled the covers over her. She flopped back on to the pillows and sighed loudly. 'Christ!' She looked at me. 'Thank you. You were very kind.'

I gave a perfunctory nod. What could I say? I didn't think I'd been kind at all. She'd had little privacy and no pain relief. I couldn't help feeling that the brutal process Sally had just gone through was in some way a perverted medical punishment for her decision to terminate the pregnancy.

'Please don't think badly of me, Nurse,' Sally begged. A petite girl with green eyes, her long dark hair was pulled back in an untidy ponytail.

I put my hand gently on the side of her face. 'I don't think badly of you, Sally. Not at all.'

'My mother has motor neurone disease,' she explained, her voice starting to tremble. 'I'm caring for her and my three younger sisters. Daddy died of heart failure a year ago. I can't bring a baby into the world, not now. I tried to protect myself. I did. I did.'

Sally burst into tears and I sat on the bed and hugged her while she sobbed into my shoulder. Guilt. Shame. Relief. Regret. She had it all.

Weeping a little myself, I realized that a woman's journey through life was defined and controlled by her ability to reproduce. It dictated what we did with our lives, and when, and it mandated our financial future unless we had the right to manage our own fertility. In England, we had won the right to have control over our bodies, but the ongoing controversy over abortion was cruelly leaving a guilty stain in many minds.

Eleanor returned to the bedside. 'It's fine,' she said. 'Everything has come out.'

Sally dried her eyes. 'Was it a boy or girl?'

'I'm not sure,' Eleanor said evasively. 'Would you like a bath or tea first?'

'Tea would be lovely.'

When Sally had finished her tea and was in the bath, I went to find Eleanor.

'Come with me,' Eleanor said.

Reluctantly I accompanied her to the sluice, knowing she was going to show me the foetus.

'Good grief,' I said, when she removed the paper cover. Lying on its side in the bedpan was the tiny foetus. It was a brownish-red colour with a head almost twice the size of the rest of it. But that wasn't the fascinating part. Clasped under the foetus's pencil-thin arm was a pink intrauterine device that had been implanted in Sally's uterus to prevent pregnancy.

'Little devil,' Eleanor said.

'What do we do with the foetus now?' I asked.

'We put it in the hospital waste for incineration.'

'Oh, how sad,' I said.

And it really was.

Later, wallowing in hot water into which I had thrown two of Tilly's rose bath cubes that she had carelessly left in our communal bathroom, my mind returned to Sally. Only a little older than me, she would be home by now looking after her sick mother and younger siblings. Preparing dinner. Washing clothes. Helping with homework.

Eleanor told me that two doctors had to sign approval for a termination, and that it was performed if the doctors considered there was a risk to the mother's physical and mental health if the pregnancy continued. Sally's decision to abort was made on the needs of her family, not her own. Having taken precautions, she had not been irresponsible. Poor girl had simply had rotten luck.

Mrs Field wasn't expected to last the night. Sister Sonya, who was visibly upset, had phoned Mrs Field's relatives to inform them that her condition had deteriorated rapidly during the afternoon.

All of the day's operations had been uneventful. Mrs Wagstaff's ovarian cyst had been removed and she would be discharged in a few days. Debra Cadogan had come through her hysterectomy with flying colours. And Mrs Barnes was also recovering well. The mass had not spread through the uterine wall and she still had her ovaries. She now had an anxious wait for pathology to determine if the mass was cancerous.

Reaching forward, I ran the hot tap again and wondered when my own turn for problems in the gynae department would come. None of us seemed to escape it.

As Sister Sonya predicted, Merrivale Field died at 9 p.m. on the evening of my first day on the ward.

The following morning, I asked Sister Sonya how she had known that death was imminent. It was a question she wasn't expecting, and it required thought.

'I think,' she said eventually, 'that it's mostly intuition and experience, but it's also blending physical signs with intangible perceptions.'

Clear as mud. I thanked her, but it would be a few years before I understood what she meant.

Mrs Barnes was discharged eight days after her operation with a clean bill of health. The mass in her uterus was luckily benign, so she didn't require any follow-up treatment. Her daughter had re-booked the church wedding for the following month, and Mrs Barnes couldn't wait to start the apricot dainties.

Hysterectomies were popular in the seventies, and the go-to operation for menopause problems, endometriosis, painful heavy periods, fibroids, uterine prolapse and cancer. It would be some time before other treatments were available, or hysterectomy would be considered as a last resort. I can't think of any of my mother's friends who hadn't had one, as had my mother.

This was Mum's take on the matter.

'Doctor, I'm having bad headaches.'

'Here, take these anti-depressants and we'll whip your womb out and you'll be fine.'

'But the problem's in my head, Doctor.'

'Precisely.'

My mother had a point. Misogyny was frequently the elephant in the room, and although most male doctors were fantastic, a few had difficulty telling the difference between an irrational woman and an emotional woman. Some even worked on the principle that if they hadn't heard of the woman's symptoms, then the illness simply didn't exist. Some still do.

A daytime glance into any hospital ward would immediately tell you if it was a male or female ward. The latter resembled flowerbeds at Kew Gardens, and while the effect looked pretty and smelt good, each bouquet needed to be removed from the ward every evening, in an appropriately labelled vase, and returned to the patient the following morning.

Usually the preserve of student nurses, this arduous but fragrant chore was supposedly undertaken to stop flowers murdering patients during the night by using up gases required for human respiration. The real reason, of course, was to stop the night nurses knocking them over in the dark. I expect the asphyxiation angle was dreamed up by the same backyard scientist who decided that all pillowcase openings should face away from the ward entrance so that dust didn't blow into the pillows.

Another way of murdering patients with flowers was the clever use of floral arrangements. Red and white flowers in the same vase signified an imminent death, and woe betide a student nurse who made such a mistake. When my own thoughtless flower-arranging caused the demise of a patient, regardless of the fact that she was ninety-two with terminal cancer, I was told by Sister Sonya that if a sparrow landed on my piano, this also forewarned of an approaching death.

'I don't know about you,' I told her, with a healthy dose of sarcasm, 'but we don't keep our piano in the garden.'

People say the resultant tongue-lashing could be heard in Aberdeen.

I enjoyed nursing the women on the gynae ward. Having spent much of their lives looking after the physical and emotional needs of others, they were appreciative of everything we nurses did for them. Many, like Mrs Barnes, had delayed seeking treatment because of family commitments – a misguided maternal benevolence that was to feature prominently in my own life in the not too distant future.

Some women were reluctant to put anyone out, while others feared being told by a doctor that their illness was of their own doing. This last was, and always will be, a major problem for early detection. What woman was going to seek help if she feared a diagnosis might be attributed to her weight, diet, contraceptive practices, pregnancy history, lack of exercise or something else that she didn't know could hurt her?

For a while, I was bothered by the ethical issues of placing women admitted for infertility or miscarriage on the same ward as women having abortions. This seemed a cruelty that I couldn't comprehend, but there was a surprising *esprit de corps* between the patients, regardless of why they were there. It was all women's business, make no mistake, and everyone got on with it as best they could.

As I walked out of Dulwich Hospital after my last day on the gynae ward, I was more than a little proud of being a woman.

CHAPTER 10

The Workhouse

St Francis Hospital, London: Early 1972

MY PARENTS HAD given me money at Christmas to buy a warm winter coat, and I was busy spending it unwisely. Hitting the January sales was the true start of the London season for those of us without a private income and a title, and I was trying on a backless dress and admiring myself in the mirror in the changing room at Biba when a hip, happening, long-haired girl wearing black leather trousers, a short fur coat and thick eyeliner asked me, 'Are you a nurse?'

I sighed. Not a week went by when I wasn't asked this question. How did she know? Was it the socks? 'Which bit gave me away?' I asked.

She shrugged and smiled. 'I don't know. You look nice, I suppose.'

Nice!

I smiled back, thinking I would give my eye teeth to look like her.

'What do *you* do?' I asked.

'I'm a rep at Rank Xerox.'

A rep at Rank Xerox! It sounded amazing.

As the girl was leaving the changing room, she

turned and said, 'Actually, if you really want to know, it was your sensible shoes that gave you away.'

'Oh,' I said despondently.

I looked down at the sensible shoes I had been forced to buy when I started nursing; shoes that had been splashed with every conceivable bodily fluid, and which I'd had to wear today as all my other pairs were wet. 'Bastards,' I said to them unkindly.

On the bus home, I clung to the bag containing the backless dress and thought about Rank Xerox. It sounded like some sort of space programme, one that required the girl to have a nuclear physics degree. Impressed, I thought about studying physics for two minutes, and then I thought about buying black leather trousers for over an hour.

Curious, I asked the Duchess of Tesco (my mother's current title) if she knew what a rep did at Rank Xerox.

'Not much,' Mum said. 'Rank Xerox make photocopy machines. A rep is just a representative who sells them.'

I nearly fell over. Was that all it was? There was a lesson in there somewhere and I was darned if I could figure out what it was. But then, at nineteen, the oddest things impressed me. I had recently been enthralled by two men dressed in overalls who had walked into King's and advised the ward sisters that they were taking the televisions in the day rooms to be serviced. Cool as can be, they loaded the televisions into a van, drove away and the televisions were never seen again.

Roy Webley had grown up with a fear of the workhouse. At the first sign of bad behaviour, his mother used to threaten him and his brother with being sent there. But Roy's good behaviour hadn't protected him for ever, and here he was, eighty-five years later, at the workhouse for the poor and destitute that he had so feared being sent to in his childhood. It didn't matter that the grim red-brick building was now called St Francis Hospital. To Roy, it was still the workhouse, and he knew he was going to die there and was as depressed as hell about it.

A proud railwayman, Roy had been a train guard and an Arsenal supporter all his life. He smoked two packets of cigarettes a day and was hugely overweight. The most exercise he'd ever had was arm-wrestling down the pub. His brother had died of liver failure and his wife, Molly, of lung cancer. His three coal-miner sons lived miles away in Newcastle upon Tyne and never visited him.

Apart from Meals on Wheels – or Muck in a Truck, as it was known in East Dulwich – there were no available community services to support Roy at home when he was diagnosed with chronic lung disease and diabetes. Unable to care for himself, he was admitted to St Francis.

The other old men on Roy's ward told a similar story of being struck down by illness and the frailties of old age. Several had fought in two wars, most were widowed, none had their own teeth or pyjamas, and many were bedridden and incontinent. They were all football mad, hated Germans, loved beer, horse-racing and cigarettes, and a few were busy setting the world on fire one bedspread at a time. Like Roy, they knew St Francis had been a workhouse and hated it. It was tragic, but that was the way it was.

I didn't want to be at St Francis either, but it was my turn to provide another three months of cheap student-nurse labour to keep the National Health Service afloat. I'd been dreading my allocation to

St Francis – the stories I'd heard made it sound more frightful than Dickens at St Giles.

But it wasn't. Despite the dreary surroundings, the terrible smell and the workhouse shadow that hovered over them, the male patients on my ward were polite, grateful and spirited at times. They were nothing like those rude old codgers on Dickens. On top of that, the regular staff had a good relationship with the patients and each other, and no one complained about the heavy workload. It was Camelot compared with Dickens, but then the ward sister, Sister Gwen, was on holiday in Blackpool. Her absence most probably explained the pleasant camaraderie among the staff.

St Francis, or Franny's, as we called it, lay on flat land on the other side of the railway line to Dulwich Hospital. A pedestrian tunnel under the line linked the two hospitals, and that was the only connection. I never saw a medical student or any of our nurse tutors at St Francis, and rarely did a doctor or a visitor appear.

That said, the care on my ward was second to none. Student nurses comprised the bulk of the staff, and we worked hard. There were no bedsores on any of the long-time residents, but there were on new patients, who were admitted after lying in bed at home for weeks, some wounds so big you could fit your fist in them. Those wounds required daily dressings and took months to heal, if they ever did.

I'd been working at St Francis for two weeks when Sister Gwen returned from Blackpool. With stoic resignation that things would now start on a downward trajectory, I thought I was prepared for Sister Gwen.

But sitting at the office desk was the stern-faced,

tank-sized, top banana who had interviewed me eighteen months ago.

Hopefully, she wouldn't remember me.

'You?' she said, when I reported on duty. 'God almighty! How come you've lasted this long?'

She remembered me all right.

Sister Gwen had numerous chins and the largest chest in the known mammalian world. You'd have had to cut her in half and count the rings to see how old she was, but I'm guessing around a hundred and five.

Although there were many notable exceptions, British hospitals in the 1970s specialized in retaining imperious, loony old nursing sisters, who took great pleasure in wielding pointless rules and being needlessly unkind to young nurses. Strongly suspecting that would be the case here, I braced myself for a torrid time. I didn't know it, but I was about to learn what a woman given a little power was truly capable of. And all of it would be good.

You see, nothing changed on the ward. The staff remained convivial, the patients were pleased to see Sister Gwen, and laughter could occasionally be heard. Unbelievably, she handed out sticks of pink-and-white Blackpool rock. Something was very wrong. Sister Gwen's benevolence had me on full alert!

It took an hour working with her for me to realize that her real persona bore no resemblance to the frightening woman who had interviewed me. A rough diamond, she smoked heavily, swore loudly and worked as hard as the rest of us. Her heart was as big as Texas, and it was her mission in life to make sure everyone was warm, clean, dry and well fed, including her nurses. Everyone adored her. And things were going to be done her way, no matter what the elusive doctors said.

Her boys (as she called the patients) received their own newspaper each morning and a pale ale in a proper beer glass on Sundays.

'It's like this, chum,' Sister Gwen told the man from the finance department, who disapproved of such largesse. 'You've gotta give my boys something to look forward to.'

There wasn't much learning happening on the ward, and Sister Gwen never had time to supervise us, but I was okay with that. I knew I should be receiving proper pay for what I was doing, but as the work didn't bother me, and because it was worthwhile, I decided to view my time at Franny's as volunteering. Which in a way it was. And I'll tell you something else. Placing the hospital budget ahead of proper clinical nurse tuition might have been bad for student-nurse training, but having efficient, hard-working student nurses caring for the old folk at Franny's was the best thing that could have happened to them. That and Sister Gwen, of course.

One elderly gent from another ward, who had all his marbles, could walk with his frame and take a taxi to the nearby bookie's, was tasked with overseeing the financial trades for the horse-racing fanatics. He took orders, placed bets and collected winnings. Known as Rapid Reg, most unexpectedly it was Reg Snape from Dickens!

We greeted each other like long-lost relatives. He had recovered from his stroke and appeared well.

'It's much better here, love,' he told me. 'People are nicer and I've got a job.'

I was happy to see him doing so well. It's amazing how much we all need a reason to get up in the morning.

A week later, on the train home to visit my parents, I was thinking about Roy Webley when I had another of my good ideas. Reg Snape told me he had worked as a fettler on the railways and I knew that Roy had been a train guard: what about bringing them together and reviving Roy's interest in trains? I couldn't wait to return to work and run the idea past Sister Gwen.

My brother and I had been mad trainspotters when we were young and had spent many summer holidays at Portchester station, our faces flushed with excitement as the Portsmouth trains sped past us. And our train obsession hadn't ended there, either. The attic room of our small house in Portchester was entirely given over to a large model train set. We talked gauges and built sheds and bridges and tunnels, and Richard even let me use his Meccano, but only the green bits.

'Bloody brilliant!' Sister Gwen said, when I told her my idea. 'That should cheer up old Roy. And they can talk trains over a beer. The poor sods don't get beer on Reg's ward.'

The inaugural railway workers' meeting was arranged for the following afternoon, and Reg turned up early. He and Roy settled in chairs and I delivered the beers. They were quiet for a time, drinking and sizing each other up.

'You see, Roy,' Reg explained eventually, 'you gotta believe this place is a railway station. Like St Pancras station, except this here's St Francis station.'

Roy didn't look convinced.

'Me,' Reg went on, 'I think I'm living in a station because I can hear trains go past. Someone brings me food and tea and I don't have to clean nothing.'

'But it's the workhouse . . .' Roy said despondently.

'No, it ain't, Roy. Has anyone asked you to crush bones for fertilizer since you've been here?'

Roy shook his head.

'Have you spiked oakum?' Reg asked, referring to the filthy workhouse job of using a nail to pick out reusable bits of rope fibres from old oakum, the tarred rope used for caulking ships.

Roy shook his head again.

'See?' Reg said with conviction. 'We've got it made, you and me!'

From then on, Reg and Roy met regularly to talk about the good old days of steam over a beer.

Two more men who had worked on the railways put up their hands for the train club. One, a mountain of a man, had worked as a fireman on the Flying Scotsman.

Yep. My brother was going to be so jealous.

During my last month at St Francis, on a lovely spring day, I was walking along the covered walkway that abutted the hospital when I noticed water pouring from under the toilet door. Often used by the public taking the short-cut under the railway line, the single toilet had a small sink and the door opened directly on to the walkway. Thinking someone had left the tap running, I tried the door, but it wouldn't open. Being a seaman's daughter and conscious of water wastage, I hurried back to the ward and told Sister Gwen, who went to find the janitor.

A short time later, a pale and shaken Sister Gwen returned to the ward. An unknown man had hanged himself from the chain attached to the lavatory cistern. The police were called and the body was taken away.

'You want a belt of something, Johnson?' Sister Gwen asked me.

'No thanks, Sister.'

'It wasn't a question,' she said forcefully, and steered me into her office.

We never learned the man's name.

Coming to terms with a patient's death was something I never mastered on the emotional spectrum. Other nurses, it seemed to me, were able to detach themselves professionally, but I always made mental connections with the bereaved and visualized the devastation a death left behind. My bigger picture was visceral and profound: I could see the lonely widower at the grocer's purchasing food for one, watch an inconsolable woman setting a single place at the kitchen table, and hear the sobbing child in the classroom while other students made Mother's Day cards.

During my first year of training, I had witnessed several deaths of elderly patients, none of which was unexpected. As autopsies or transplant protocols were not required, and rarely were unusual cultural practices to be observed, ward nurses prepared the body for the mortuary or the undertaker, the latter often collecting bodies directly from the ward at St Francis.

To help me cope with the cold, clinical process of performing last offices for a patient I had known in life, I undertook a personal metamorphosis. It would begin as the curtains were pulled around the death bed to allow the body to repose for an hour and the soul supposedly to float off to Heaven. By the time I had prepared the mortuary pack, filled in labels to be attached to a foot and covered my uniform with a hospital gown, my own transformation was complete.

I had turned into my mother . . .

I have a clear memory of when I was about four years old and our neighbour, Mrs Saunders, leaned over the back fence that separated our gardens, parted the snowy cascade of Michaelmas daisies on our side with her hands and frantically called out to my mother, 'Marion! Marion! Harold won't wake up!'

Harold Saunders's was the first dead body I ever saw. Forgotten in the melee, I followed my mother next door and observed the goings-on from the Saunderses' bedroom doorway.

'I'm so sorry, but Harold's gone,' I heard Mum say. Mrs Saunders gasped and buried her face in her hands.

Mesmerized, I watched as my mother removed the old man's pillow from under his head and laid him flat. Gently, she closed his eyes with her fingers and pushed some teeth that were in a glass on the bedside table into his mouth. She positioned one of Mr Saunders's ties under his chin and tied it tightly in a bow on top of his head. I would later discover this was to keep his false teeth in place and his mouth closed while rigor mortis set in. Then she put a penny on each closed eye and pulled the sheet up over his face before calling the doctor.

I didn't see another dead body until I was a student nurse and it was my turn to tie bows on top of heads, exactly like my mother had done, albeit using bandages instead of ties. I have no idea how my mother knew what to do in the event of a death, although the knowledge was almost certainly a souvenir of war. It was my mother's capable and controlled actions at

Harold Saunders's bedside that I would call upon many times in later years. I'd remember Mrs Saunders leaning over our back fence and parting the Michaelmas daisies. I would think of her elderly husband, Harold, and how he had died peacefully in his own jimjams at home in his sleep. And I would whisper, 'Way to go, Harold. Way to go.'

One afternoon, Sister Gwen and I were cleaning up after performing last offices on our third deceased elderly gentleman that weekend – more often than not, deaths occurred in threes. As a mark of respect, we rarely spoke during these solemn procedures, and I suppose it was only natural that afterwards we scrubbed our hands until they were raw.

I was still rinsing death away when Sister Gwen shook water off her hands and turned to face me.

'Okay, Maggie Johnson,' she said. 'Who the fuck's this Harold bloke?'

On my last day at St Francis, Sister Gwen had tea and cake waiting in the office, as she always did for students moving on to their next ward.

'You know, Johnson,' she said to me candidly, 'I was worried that I'd made a big mistake letting you start training. I thought you were a spoiled, privileged pain in the arse, but you've proved me wrong. I expect we all misjudge people. You probably had me all wrong too.'

'No, Sister,' I said. 'I thought you were wonderful right from the start.'

Always leave them smiling.

CHAPTER 11

The Teapot of Life

King's College Hospital, London: Summer 1972

BY THE BEGINNING of June, I had completed over half of
my training and was ready to move out of the nurses'
home. A few girls preferred the security of remaining
at the hospital, but the rest of us left skid marks on the
way out of the door.

Over the next couple of years, I lived in a succession
of large Victorian terrace houses in Herne Hill, not far
from King's. There were numerous such houses in the
neighbourhood occupied by nurses and medical
students, and my friends and I migrated like swallows
in and out of premises in Hollingbourne Road,
Holmdene Avenue and Beckwith Road.

Courtesy of the Thames Basin, the houses had an
air of aching dampness about them, with mouldy
wallpaper, peeling plaster and threadbare carpet. Some
had a coin box on the wall for electricity, and a gas hot-
water heater over the bath. Mood lighting was generously
provided by bare bulbs hung from the ceiling.

Jan, Kathy and I tended to share houses with three
or four male students, mostly medical but some studying
law or chemistry. We girls usually lived on the ground

floor and the boys upstairs, and we formed strong friendships, irritated the hell out of each other, made mistakes, squabbled over cleaning and food in the fridge, then apologized and made up later down the pub.

Faced with a less than salubrious canvas, we appointed the common areas in our houses with fridges that belonged in a museum, stolen street signs, junk-shop furniture, posters, guitars, bicycles and the world's loudest stereo systems. Hardly anyone owned a car, but as there was no off-street parking, this was an advantage in a way – although Kathy always managed to find a spot for her red scooter.

In our own rooms, we girls specialized in bohemian chic and made brick-and-plank bookcases, built modular display cabinets with wooden orange boxes, and festooned our beds and windows with paisley-print fabrics. We papered our walls with avant-garde posters, installed Tiffany lampshades over the bulbs, and burned incense and scented candles on saucers. Talk about styling.

Money was an ever-present worry when living out. After rent and necessities, there was little left over, and to avoid starvation I joined the nurses who covertly dined in the ward kitchens on untouched meals that had been delivered to patients who couldn't eat. Usually famished, we stood between open cupboard doors in the kitchen and hastily ate off a shelf, ready to close the doors and calmly step away from the crime scene if a ward sister walked in: being caught meant instant dismissal.

Laundry was also a problem once we had moved out. The hospital continued to launder our uniforms, but no longer took our clothes, sheets and towels. We didn't have a washing machine, so we loaded our dirty washing into a hot, soapy bath and stomped up and down on everything while listening to the Beach Boys (they were our washing music). We drained the bath, refilled it with cold water and stomped some more until our feet turned blue. We dried things outside, on racks in our rooms, and with a hairdryer if an item was urgently required.

Along with world-class hangovers, music was a common bond, and we played everything at full volume, sometimes different albums blasting from different rooms. My musical tastes were eclectic. I had grown up listening to the Swedish tenor Jussi Björling, Bizet's *Carmen*, Bach's liturgical music, *South Pacific* and Arthur Rubinstein playing Liszt, and my early teenage years were filled with Elvis, The Hollies, Manfred Mann and the Beatles. In more recent years, I had graduated to the Stones, David Bowie, The Who, Led Zeppelin and Santana, but now the Eagles, Neil Young, Carole King, Cat Stevens and James Taylor were cruising into prime position. Missing the classics, a couple of times I walked around the outside of the Albert Hall, admiring the bright red Fareham bricks and wondering how I could ever afford a ticket to a performance.

It remains one of the great mysteries of my London years how we could afford to do anything at all. Impoverished students, we somehow managed to major in the five basic food groups: beer, gin, fish, chips and Chinese takeaway. I never once saw anyone take illegal drugs, or knew of anyone who took them. We were all far too busy drinking and having sex.

'Look out, Mike. Here she comes,' Dennis called, as I walked down the middle of Twining ward at King's. I was wearing stout wellington boots and carrying a bucket of warm, soapy water, a funnel and a long rubber tube.

'That will do, thank you, Dennis,' I said curtly. Dennis was a bus conductor immobilized in traction after rupturing his spleen and fracturing both legs and his pelvis in a car accident.

'You're in for a thorough rogering, Mike,' Martin yelled, as I passed his bed.

'That's enough, Martin,' I said sharply. Martin was lying flat after spinal surgery. He was a bank teller who had helped a friend carry a piano up three flights of stairs.

'Are you and Mike available for children's parties?' joked Andrew, who was in the bed next to Mike's.

'Behave yourself, Andrew,' I said gruffly. Andrew was a builder and ten days post-op after complicated surgery to repair his broken collarbone, wrist, right tibia, femur and smashed patella. He had fallen from scaffolding on to a cement mixer and was lucky to be alive.

Smiling wanly at Mike, I put down the bucket and pulled the curtains around his bed. Poor Mike. Only eighteen, he had crashed his motorcycle in Streatham two weeks ago. He had stitches in his head, his right leg was in traction, two ribs were cracked, five teeth had been knocked out, and his plastered right arm was suspended from an overhead frame. It would be a while before he was released into the wild.

Often, patients who'd had major surgery and were bed-bound required enemas to help things along, and I was experienced enough to see the funny side of the taunts and jeers, but young Mike was dying of embarrassment. The curtains wouldn't afford him much privacy, and I knew there was worse to come. The lads hadn't even started doing sound effects and making comments about the smell yet.

'They only tease the men who will walk out of

here,' I told Mike, as I lifted off the traction weights, gently rolled him a little on his left side and eased a plastic sheet under him.

'Get on with it, then,' Mike said testily. His constipation had got the better of his usual pleasant demeanour.

'This takes two,' I said. 'Rosie will be here soon.'

Rosie O'Brien, now a kipper, had finally escaped the geriatric wards and, much to my delight, had started on Twining. Shortly, she appeared through the curtains and handed me a plastic apron to put on. Then she said hello to Mike and made his pillows more comfortable. Her movements were as elegant and seamless as I remembered.

'Bucket or tube?' I asked Rosie.

'Bucket,' she said, and grinned.

I greased the tube and gently inserted it into Mike's anus. 'Try and hold on to the fluid as long as you can,' I told him.

'Guess who I'm engaged to!' Rosie said, as she picked up the bucket.

I had the funnel ready for the soapy water and she started to pour it in. I had grated Fairy soap into the water and added a little turpentine for good measure.

'Dr Freeman, the houseman from Dickens?' I guessed. There had been a notable shift in the ruling that student nurses were not allowed to train if they were married, and it seemed to be a change that was naturally evolving with the times rather than a revocation of an existing regulation.

Rosie gave an uninhibited happy laugh. 'Yes!' She put down the bucket and pulled a gold chain from under her collar. Dangling from it was a sapphire engagement ring.

'Isn't it gorgeous?' Rosie gushed proudly, and quickly tucked it back under her collar.

'It's lovely, Rosie,' I said. 'Congratulations!'

'Are you still going out with Kip?' she asked, lifting up the bucket and pouring more water into the funnel.

I nodded.

'Maybe Kip will propose,' Rosie said encouragingly.

I smiled, but I really wanted to scream that I wasn't going to throw away my youth and career on an indoctrinated ideal that marriage was my destiny.

'When you ladies have quite finished!' Mike exclaimed loudly.

The silence that followed was broken by Andrew in the next bed parroting a Dalek voice: 'Evacuate, evacuate . . .'

'The other man's arse is always cleaner, eh, Mike?' Dennis yelled from the other end of the ward.

'And you can shut up an' all,' Mike shouted back at him.

Thirty minutes later, Mike was a new man, and Rosie went to fetch him a cup of tea and a biscuit.

'Right, who's next?' I demanded, as I emerged from the curtains with the bucket and rubber tubing. Those who were able pulled sheets over their heads and the rest played dead.

I was enjoying my time on Twining, and despite the seriousness of the patients' injuries and post-operative conditions, there was a positive and playful atmosphere on the ward. Named in honour of the tea merchant Richard Twining, it was a busy male orthopaedic and trauma ward. The work was physically demanding, with a lot of lifting and turning of patients who were bed-bound, and pressure care for those who had to remain flat. There was a shiny new hoist in the bathroom, although it was rarely employed, as there never seemed to be enough time to wheel it to a bedside and work out how to use the jolly thing.

In addition to pre- and post-operative care and pain control, there was considerable wound management on Twining, and a lot of basic nursing care was required, particularly for those with spinal injuries, amputations or plaster casts, and those confined to bed with complex traction attached to their limbs. This meant nurses attending to the personal needs of fully conscious young men who were temporarily incapacitated. I bed-bathed and shaved many men my own age, helped them eat and drink, held their manhood and the urinal while they peed, and wiped their behinds. I even rolled their cigarettes. Such dependence on a nurse creates a special bond, and the closeness could be challenging. But it was never dull, and definitely not a career path for a shrinking violet.

Trauma patients tended to be in hospital for a long time, and I came to know well the men I was caring for. I looked forward to seeing them and relished that the doctors and other healthcare providers visited fleetingly, and that it was nurses who maintained a constant vigil. We knew how they were and where they were at any time of day. We knew what had happened to them and what might happen to them. We knew what to watch out for and what needed to be done if something went wrong. And it was our responsibility to keep them safe and help them to recover as best they could.

On Twining, the last vestiges of my youthful self-obsession were slowly slipping away. I was starting to consider the needs of others before my own, and to anticipate those needs – a noble transformation that revealed itself when it became apparent that I couldn't wait to get to work the next day. Truly, it's a rare and beautiful thing when an unrealized passion and a career come together. I loved nursing. And nursing was finally loving me back.

My brother called late one warm summer evening to tell me that he had asked his girlfriend, Esther Stevenson, to marry him. A slender, dark-eyed beauty, Esther was a British Airways air hostess and I adored her. The wedding was to take place in Durham the following summer, a few days before my twenty-first birthday. My mother was turning cartwheels with happiness. The son she had nurtured back from the brink of death was meeting another of life's milestones: he was getting married. She was already naming the children.

I hadn't seen Richard since February, when Jan and I had hitched up north to visit him, but we had kept in contact by phone. He was busy working as a physician at the Royal Victoria Infirmary in Newcastle and learning to fly. It had long been a dream of his to become a flying doctor in Australia, but a few weeks after he gained his pilot's licence he was refused an Australian immigration visa due to his poor health. It was a setback, but he picked himself up and set about climbing the Munros in Scotland and the medical ladder of the National Health Service in England. I was pleased he wasn't going to Australia. I couldn't imagine who in their right mind would want to go there.

Our shared houses in London were always on the King's party circuit – noisy affairs that were strangely competitive in how many people turned up, how late the party finished and how many times the police were called. Invitation was by word of mouth or an invite posted on a hospital noticeboard. The hosts never knew who was coming or how many.

Owing to our late work hours, hospital parties didn't kick off until after ten, and by the time guests started to amble in, anxious hosts who had feared a flop might have passed out on a bed, often to wake later under a pile of coats.

Partygoers supplied their own booze and put cans and bottles in the bar, which was the bath filled with cold water. The hosts supplied the music, often securing the services of the incomparable disc jockey Dave, one of the doctors at King's. Peanuts and crisps (another host contribution) were tipped into bowls, and guests were discouraged from flicking ash on to the floor by the strategic placing of ashtrays made by dental students from pink plaster moulds of false teeth. Take it from me, no one could touch us for event management.

Divesting ourselves of the stress and intensity of the human dramas that filled our days, we drank and danced and loved and laughed while Roxy Music, Jimi Hendrix, Rod Stewart and the Stones blared out of our windows.

Invariably a neighbour called the police and members of the constabulary arrived in a panda car. A shining example of British taxpayers' money at work, the police would politely ask for the music to be turned down and we would comply – until they had gone and we turned it up again. Usually the police officers returned to join the party when their shift had finished.

Often, if the company and music were good, we would party all night. I lost count of the number of times I went straight from a party to work on an early duty. I have a clear recollection of sitting on stairs with Kip watching the dawn break through the open front door of a house in Hollingbourne Road, knowing that I had only half an hour to race home and put my uniform on. We were arguing about whether it was Bilbo Baggins or Bilbo Buggins, as you do at six in the morning, until Kip pointed out that there was a cigarette end floating in the white plastic beaker of wine I'd been holding for show for the past five hours. I never went to work drunk, but sometimes I was bleary-eyed from lack of sleep.

The spooky Dr Wolfbane re-entered my life by way of the letterbox in our front door at Holmdene Avenue. He had discovered my address and started sending notes describing things he could do with me, and to me. He didn't sign his name, but I recognized his scrawl from the notes he had passed me on Pantia Ralli.

Cleverly, he hadn't made threats or implied anything violent. It was a bit like the Guitano wandering-hands situation – totally creepy but nothing specific I could act upon.

A couple of days after delivery of another fruity note, I arrived home following a late duty at King's to find Wolfbane in the upstairs sitting room, chatting with one of my housemates, Ed. Ed was a tall, tanned and toned Californian, studying medicine at King's. He was sitting in an armchair, drinking from a bottle of milk. I think Ed lived on apples and milk.

'Ah, there you are,' Wolfbane said, when he saw me. He smiled, stood up and kissed me on the cheek as if we were old friends. Then he sat down.

Frozen to the spot, I flashed a look at Ed, who said, 'I'll make you a coffee, Maggie.' Alarmingly, he disappeared off to the kitchen.

I couldn't think of anything to say. My brain closed down. Along with my mouth and legs.

I could hear Wolfbane telling me that we could have a late supper in Knightsbridge and go to a hotel if I wished. His confidence was astonishing.

I just stared at him.

'Did you get my letters?' he asked.

I didn't answer.

'Not talking is silly, and it won't deter me,' he said, irritated.

I shuddered.

Ed re-entered the room and handed me a mug of coffee. I couldn't believe he had made it so quickly.

'Don't you think you should leave us alone?' Wolfbane suggested to Ed, man to man.

'Nope, I live here,' Ed said indignantly, and sat down.

Relieved, I asked Wolfbane, 'How did you know where I lived?'

'You're very cute,' Wolfbane said, ignoring my question. He turned to Ed. 'Isn't she cute? What do you think?'

Ed sat forward in the chair, rested his elbows on his knees and said quite menacingly, 'I think you should leave.'

Wolfbane laughed awkwardly, then huffed loudly. In the strangled silence that followed, he must have worked out that he was no match for Captain America, because he stood up and walked out. I don't think I breathed properly until I heard the front door slam.

Ed got up, led me over to the sofa and sat me down.

'Don't drink that coffee,' he said. 'I made it with tap water so I could come back quicker.'

I looked up at him. 'How did you know?'

'The look on your face when I left the room.'

Terrified that Wolfbane would return and one of my other housemates might accidentally let him in, I spent the night on Ed's bed. We top-and-tailed, and there was no hanky-panky. After a while, a small voice in the dark asked, 'Am I cute, Ed?'

'No, Maggie, you are definitely not cute,' a husky voice answered.

'Thank goodness,' I said and smiled. Ed was such a glorious musketeer.

About a month after Wolfbane had visited the house, another note arrived from him. This one was a foul, name-calling, disgusting thing. I showed it to Jan, then burned it. Wolfbane never bothered me again, but I can still see the words in that note.

Years later, I was watching an old Hitchcock movie on television when I suddenly realized who Wolfbane had reminded me of. It was Norman Bates, the nutter in *Psycho*.

Archibald Leach, also known as Arson Archie, was admitted to Twining with a broken arm and a broken leg, injuries he had reportedly sustained by falling from his bunk at Brixton Prison. Seventy-eight years old and weighing only eight stone, Archie fancied himself as a ladies' man and had been married four times. He came accessorized with two burly prison warders.

The warders, Mick and Stan (whom Archie referred to as Tweeledum and Tweedledee), stood outside the operating theatre while Archie's arm and leg were repaired under general anaesthetic and full plaster casts were fitted to both limbs. They escorted him back to the ward, handcuffed his good arm to the bedrail and sat one each side of his bed. Their prisoner was in full view of the entire ward and had as much chance of escaping as Rudolf Hess had from Spandau Prison in Berlin. The other patients thought that so much security for a frail old man was a criminal waste of taxpayers' money.

'Isn't old Archie in prison for arson?' I asked Stan.

Stan grinned. 'Yep.'

'Then why does he need *two* warders?'

'Because he set fire to his wives,' Mick said, and I gulped back an inappropriate snigger.

'But he can't move and we can all see him,' I reasoned.

Mick agreed and telephoned the prison. It was decided that as long as Archie was handcuffed to the bed, one warder was enough.

It wasn't. After Mick had returned to Brixton Prison, and while Stan was reading the paper, Archie took the thermometer from the wall holder above his bed and forced it down his own throat. Needless to say, emergency surgery was required to remove it.

Rather proud to have nursed a dangerous prisoner, on my next visit home I was relating the story of seventy-eight-year-old Archie Leach to my mother when she interrupted me. 'He's not seventy-eight, you know. He's only sixty-eight.'

'Who is?' I asked.

'Cary Grant,' she replied.

'What's Cary Grant got to do with it?'

'You don't know?' my mother questioned.

'Know what?' I said.

'Archie Leach is Cary Grant's real name. Your prisoner was using it as an alias. Wasn't that the point of your story?'

I smiled at my mother. 'Of course it was,' I agreed.

'Liar,' she shot back. 'You had no idea.'

'Did so . . .'

As an experienced second-year student nurse, I was gaining more responsibility on the ward, at times with a first-year student nurse under my wing.

It was also about this time that nurses were starting to return to the workforce after having raised a family. Encouraged by the women's movement to revive their careers, qualified staff nurses in their late thirties and early forties were reappearing on the wards. Understandably, they were nervous about their lack of knowledge of new drugs and procedures, and quite at a loss with some of the equipment. Rosie and I found ourselves in the odd situation of explaining things to senior nurses, and I think this made Rosie feel more confident about her training. It certainly did me.

It amused us that the older staff nurses, having trained in what Rosie and I thought of as the dark ages, were terrified of talking to doctors. Although the medics were still seen by many as demigods, well-trained nurses were starting to assert their position as the patient's protector. Day by day, we were becoming more confident about suggesting treatments and reporting concerns to medical staff.

Indeed there were times on some wards, I have to

say, when doctors, especially the new ones, were rather scared of the staff nurses and sisters.

That summer, my father, Captain Johnson, decided to hang up his sextant and retire from a life at sea. He had joined the British Merchant Navy in his mid-teens and transferred to the Royal Navy during the Second World War. Torpedoed twice, and saved both times after drifting for days in an open lifeboat, he had returned to the Merchant Navy at the end of the war, joined Esso and become a master mariner.

My mother was anxious about having Herbie J permanently around the house so she tarted up the workshop area in the garage and drafted long to-do lists to keep him busy. But she needn't have worried. My father's to-do list for her was longer. And quite different.

Having spent most of their married life apart, my father set about romancing my mother and showered her with jewels, affection and attention. They played golf, cycled through the beautiful South Downs, walked hand in hand along the beach at Swanage, flew to Aruba for holidays in the sun, and kept Gordon's gin and the British racing industry in business.

It was an idyllic time for them, which was fortuitous, as the year ahead was to be my mother's swansong.

CHAPTER 12

Nights of the Long Table

King's College Hospital, London: Autumn 1972

I WAS STANDING in the afternoon sunshine on the fore-court at the British Museum, queuing with friends to see King Tutankhamun, the golden boy with the handsome death mask. I was supposed to be working a late duty on Annie Zunz, a female medical ward at King's, but I was desperate to see Tutankhamun and had called in sick so I could tag along with friends to the exhibition.

There was a tap on my shoulder.

'Feeling better?' a voice said.

I spun around and stifled a gasp. The sister in charge of the nurses' sick bay at King's, Sister Lena, was standing behind me. And she wasn't smiling. She must have been appraised early that morning of who had called in sick.

'Yes, thank you, Sister,' I managed, and turned away. I could feel her eyes boring into the back of my head. At that moment, I knew what people meant when they said that their blood ran cold. Mine had gone glacial. Miranda and Polly, who were on genuine days off, exchanged worried looks. I'd been caught . . . and this could mean dismissal.

162

I wasn't sure what to do. Should I offer to pay for Sister Lena to see the exhibition? Run away? Faint? She had easily recognized me as I had been in sick bay a couple of times with high fever and a sore throat following my initial bout of glandular fever. It was too late to pretend I was my own identical twin. Maybe if I behaved as though nothing was wrong she might think she had made a mistake.

The queue shuffled forward a few steps and there was another, firmer, tap on my shoulder. Nervously, I turned around again.

'There is no point acting as if this isn't happening, and no point me making you report on duty now,' Sister Lena said crossly, 'but you will report on duty tomorrow and advise the ward sister that you will work your next day off to make up for the sick day.'

'Yes, Sister,' I said meekly. 'Should I . . . should I explain why?' I was a little confused. How bad was this going to be?

Sister Lena looked thoughtful. 'I don't think so,' she said at length. 'If I'd caught you shopping, you'd be in real trouble, but as this is . . . Tutankhamun, you can say you felt better in the afternoon and went out and you wish to make up the sick day.'

'Thank you, Sister,' I said gratefully.

She floored me with a conspiratorial grin. 'Don't do it again.'

I shook my head. 'I won't.'

And I didn't. I'd been a fool. I should have known that if I called in sick and went to the most popular place in London I would be caught. I was let off lightly, but the incident, I was sure, would come back to bite me later.

*

It had been quite a summer in the romance department.

My fickle heart had fallen for a dashing medical registrar at King's called Alistair. He was paged to my ward to see a patient, and our eyes had locked over a twenty-stone Turkish woman with an inflamed gall bladder. It doesn't get more romantic than that.

Kip was very cross with me, but I wasn't too cross with myself. It was only right that I allowed other British maidens to have full and unfettered access to Kip. Handsome as hell and with a wicked, sexy smile, he was a warm, compassionate and humble man, and very aware of the privilege of his King's training. One day, somewhere on this great planet of ours, I knew there would be a very lucky Mrs Kip.

Autumn leaves started falling while I was on Annie Zunz, and the approach of winter did nothing to brighten my working day. After the busy and at times playful environment on Twining, I had immediately found the heavy and laboured atmosphere on Annie Zunz stifling. With many patients elderly, overweight and bedridden by chronic illness, medical wards were always the most physically and mentally demanding to work on. For most nurses, I think.

Annie Zunz ward was said to be haunted, and at night mischievous wags would sometimes hurl a heavy wet cloth at the window to scare nurses. The cloth would thud against the window hard enough to catch your attention, then stick to the glass long enough for you to imagine an ugly grey face before it dropped off. I know this because someone did it to me, and I screamed, waking up half the ward. Naturally, I blamed the nearest patient and quickly pulled the curtain around her bed so that no one could see she was still asleep.

'It's okay,' I said loudly. 'You're just having a bad dream.'

During meal breaks on night duty at King's, we pulled our warm capes around our shoulders and took the long and silent walk through the hospital's deserted corridors to the enormous, church-like refectory on the ground floor. Most of the hospital staff were asleep in their beds, and because there were so few nurses in the refectory at night, we sat together at the long table near the kitchen. And we talked.

By day, we considered ourselves attached to our wards and had little idea what was happening elsewhere in the hospital. At night, things were different. Not only did we shoulder more responsibility on our own wards, but we also became part of the bigger hospital picture. There was a tangible night-time fellowship and we knew what was happening across the hospital.

We usually had a number of West Indian agency staff nurses and enrolled nurses working in the hospital at night, each one with a story about other hospitals where they worked. It was a staff nurse from Barbados who told me that chewing a coffee bean and having a whiff of oxygen would perk me up if I was feeling sleepy, sometimes a problem if you were sitting next to a small lamp in the middle of a dark ward while patients snored and slumbered fitfully in the shadows.

If anyone at the long table was working on Annie Zunz, the conversation soon turned to ghost stories. And that was how I learned of an amazing incident on another ward at King's – an exorcism, of all things!

I was sceptical. Friends of mine had worked on the ward and knew nothing of it, but I was assured by night nurses at our midnight meal that it had really occurred. They also told me that we were not supposed to reveal this information outside the hospital. I imagine that spilling the beans now will not be a problem.

There had been a few unexpected deaths on the ward concerned and reports from night nurses that, in the morning, empty beds appeared to have been slept on, with visible depressions in the pillows. Apparently, something needed to be done. Patients were transferred to other wards and a priest was summoned. The nurse relating the story had not personally witnessed the exorcism, neither had anyone at the long table, but they had all been reliably informed that a priest in black robes had entered the ward chanting prayers and swinging a smoking thurible.

I'd like to have seen that – if it really happened.

CHAPTER 13

The Little Dears

Belgrave Hospital for Children, London: Late 1972

AFTER I HAD passed the October block exams and earned my third-year kipper hat, I was sent to the Belgrave Hospital for Children. Like Dulwich, St Giles and St Francis hospitals, the much smaller Belgrave was also part of King's College Hospital Group. An imposing Victorian red-brick building near the Oval cricket ground, it had a small Casualty for emergency admissions, an operating theatre where minor operations were performed, and a few light and airy wards with separate glass-walled nursery rooms for babies or children who were infectious. Major surgical cases and children requiring specialist treatment were admitted to Princess Elizabeth children's ward at King's.

Most sick children were in and out of the Belgrave within a week – particularly those with croup, asthma, whooping cough, pneumonia, influenza, high fevers, dehydration, diarrhoea and vomiting, convulsions and minor operations – and there were always disadvantaged children with bad colds, tapeworm, scabies, impetigo and infected sores that GPs felt should be hospitalized to ensure their recovery. There were also several

167

long-term regulars who had spent much of their young lives in hospital – children with bowel disorders, neurological problems, complications from birth injuries, cerebral palsy, endocrine disorders and blood diseases such as sickle-cell anaemia, which affected the growing West Indian population in the area.

While it wasn't Narnia, every effort had been made to make the wards at the Belgrave attractive. The heart of my ward had iron cots and beds around the outside walls and a play area in the middle with toys and games. On the walls above the cots were pretty tiles depicting nursery rhymes, and during quiet times nurses told the children stories to match the tiles – except I was naughty and never told the traditional stories. And to set the record straight, Little Bo Peep was not the butcher's daughter and she didn't have a dog called Mint Sauce.

In 1972, the much-awaited Briggs Report into the quality and nature of the professional training required for nurses and midwives was published. Like many student nurses, I hoped it would address our concerns that we were used as cheap labour in difficult-to-staff hospital facilities where no relevant teaching or training supervision was taking place.

And it did!

In a shocking revelation, Professor Asa Briggs announced to the completely uninterested populace that current nurse training in the United Kingdom was inadequate, and stated the need for a large expansion of student training and teaching. He made recommendations that more professional tutors should be placed on wards to improve teaching in clinical settings, and that qualified nurses and midwives should receive increased professional training.

Briggs also outlined that considerable emphasis should be placed on training students of high academic ability (this was already in place at London teaching hospitals, with the preference for students with three A levels). Moreover, he recommended that education structures and integrated career paths for nurses and midwives be established, and that research into nursing be pursued in conjunction with universities.

Being realists, my friends and I were not holding our breath over any of it: every nurse in the country knew that the Treasury and hospital administrators would oppose any reforms that increased the cost of training nurses and risked the hospitals losing student labour on the wards.

And we were right. It would take many years for Briggs's recommendations to be adopted. Why? Because men were in charge of the finances, women made up the bulk of the nursing workforce, and money was the bottom line.

By the end of 1972, there was a little positive action on the money front. Inflation in Britain was running high and there was widespread industrial action by many workers. Watching from the sidelines, we student nurses were too scared to march or to voice our feelings openly – although formal warnings were never made, there were intimidating rumours that nurses would suffer consequences if we caused embarrassment to the hospital. So we kept quiet.

We had, however, been modestly militant in another way, if you can call writing letters militant. When I started training in 1970, the Raise the Roof campaign, spearheaded by the Royal College of Nursing, had involved the national distribution of a campaign letter demanding better pay for nurses – a letter that people were encouraged to sign and forward to the health secretary. The government had duly received a million letters of support from across the country, including from my mother. By 1972, this campaign had finally achieved a salary increase of twenty-two per cent, which sounds fantastic but then twenty-two per cent of hardly anything is . . . let's see . . . hardly anything.

There are two things in a hospital that no amount of clinical neutrality, ward experience or classroom training can prepare you for, and they are called twins: in this instance, the utterly scrumptious red-headed Angus and Lachlan Cavendish, aged three and newly arrived in the Big Smoke from bonny Scotland. I wanted to steal both of them.

Angus was the older by seven minutes, but significantly smaller and less robust than his brother. He'd been complaining of pain in his right leg since falling the day before on to grass. His concerned parents, who had not had time to find anywhere to live in London and register with a general practitioner, had brought Angus into Casualty where X-rays revealed a fractured tibia (shinbone) in his right leg.

A broken bone from an insignificant fall was unusual, and the Casualty doctor questioned Mrs Cavendish in depth, in particular about the boy's frail condition compared with that of his brother.

Mrs Cavendish told an all too familiar tale of ignored maternal concerns. Many times over the past year, she had reported to her general practitioner that something was wrong with Angus, that since he had turned two he was not growing like Lachlan, that he was grizzly, that he wouldn't eat properly and that he often complained of tummy aches. Mrs Cavendish had also requested a referral to a paediatrician, but was told by her GP that she was overly anxious, that Angus's tummy aches were attention-seeking, and that he was just going through a slow growth phase and would catch up.

But Mrs Cavendish had not been placated, and when Mr Cavendish, a detective, had accepted a job at Scotland Yard, she had planned to find a GP in London who would believe her and refer Angus to a specialist. While unfortunate, Angus's fall was propitious in that help was now immediately available.

In Casualty, a plaster cast was applied to Angus's broken leg from his ankle to just above his knee, and he was admitted to the Belgrave for investigations. It was deemed unnecessarily stressful to separate the Cavendish twins, so Lachlan was admitted as well. The Casualty doctor had written in capital letters across the top of the admission form: ALWAYS LISTEN TO THE MOTHER.

The twins were housed in large cots in a nursery room where we could see them through the glass at all times. We tied the cots side by side so the mattresses were flush, and we lowered the inside rails to form one big cot so the boys could be properly together – an important consideration for Angus.

There was keen competition among the nurses over which of us would care for the twins, and I was a shoo-in because I had worked much of the past week in the milk kitchen, preparing large numbers of feeding bottles – one of the most disliked jobs on the ward.

Angus was fragile, weak and frightened, and a little dopey from medication to control his pain. For several days, he lay in the cot looking wan while Lachlan sat beside him and held his hand with a worried look on his face. Angus hadn't spoken a word since admission, not even in response to Lachlan's constant chatter. At first, I thought my inability to understand what Lachlan was saying was because of his strong Glasgow (Glazghee) accent, but I was wrong. Between them, the twins had developed a peculiar language that was fascinating and private.

While providing full nursing care to Angus, I encouraged Lachlan to leave the cot and play with the toys and other children on the ward, but he wasn't having it. If I tried to move him, he would grab Angus's arm and scream, so I gave up on that idea. Lachlan was, however, immediately enthralled by the paediatrician, Dr Rabjones, who pretended that Lachlan was Angus and the plaster cast was on the wrong twin.

'I'll have a word with that Casualty doctor,' Dr Rabjones said. 'He came in a box of cornflakes, so I'm not surprised.'

A short, avuncular man with a ready smile and a winning way with nurses, patients and their parents, if ever a doctor was suited to his speciality it was Rabjones, but even he couldn't entice Angus to talk. Everyone was worried the illness and trauma had caused a severe emotional response.

Dr Rabjones looked to me for feedback and I shook my head. 'Angus hasn't spoken a word to anyone since he was admitted.'

Smiling at Angus, Dr Rabjones said, 'I see.' Fumbling in his pocket, he took out a pen and drew a rabbit on Angus's plaster cast.

Angus took no notice and stared at the ceiling.

Because of his short stature, Dr Rabjones had to stand on the stool in order to perch on the cot beside Angus, and when he had done so he rolled up his trouser leg and drew another rabbit on his own knee.

Lachlan demanded, 'Me too,' and a rabbit was drawn on Lachlan's knee. Thankfully I was wearing black stockings.

Suddenly Sister appeared in the doorway. 'Off the bed, please, Doctor,' she ordered crossly. He jumped off and saluted her.

And then Angus laughed. He actually laughed!

'That's wonderful,' Sister trilled, and the consultant winked at me.

Angus was diagnosed with rickets, a disease of early childhood caused by vitamin D deficiency. It resulted in soft bones, fractures and skeletal deformities, and there was already a slight bowing of Angus's legs. His treatment was bed rest, vitamin D and calcium supplements. Caught at this stage, there was every chance his mild limb deformities would straighten out and he would completely recover.

I had not seen rickets before, but I knew of it. It was a feared disease with much social stigma attached to it when I was growing up in Britain in the 1950s, and mothers were encouraged to dose their children with cod liver oil as a preventive measure. Once a week, before school, my mother had given Richard and me a spoonful of the repulsive-tasting liquid.

On cod liver oil days, after we had waved goodbye

and Mum had closed the front door, I vomited over the Saunderses' garden wall, breakfast included. Richard, who could graze on dog biscuits and hard green blackberries, walked me down the hill to the back door of the Portsdown Inn, where he secured a glass of milk for his hungry sister. After drinking the milk and thanking the publican, we caught the school bus down to the village. A by-product of those cod liver oil days was that for years I thought men went to the pub to drink milk.

The cause of Angus's rickets was more of a concern. Why did he have a vitamin D deficiency? As both twins were raised with the same food and in the same environment, it was apparent that the usual causes of rickets – malnutrition and lack of sunlight – were not the culprits in Angus's case. A disorder of the intestines was suspected. The relevant specialist was summoned, and coeliac disease was diagnosed. The inflammation in Angus's intestine had prevented proper absorption of vitamin D, and thus induced the rickets. His treatment was supplemented with a special diet that included lots of eggs and fish (and no wheat products) to address both the rickets and the coeliac disease.

At mealtimes, I put both boys' meals on a tray between them on the mattress, and I quickly noticed that Lachlan wouldn't touch his food until Angus had finished his. Lachlan then swapped plates and tried to make Angus eat his meal too. How sweet was that? I solved the problem by ordering an extra meal for an imaginary patient called Captain Rickets and gave three meals to the twins.

'Angus likes concerned milk when he's sad,'

Lachlan said to me one morning, after Angus had refused breakfast and was a little teary. Hiding my amusement, I put some condensed milk into a bottle and made a larger hole in the teat so Angus could lie down and drink it.

Angus ailed for two weeks, then rallied to make a rapid physical recovery, but he still wasn't speaking. Not even to Lachlan. He was on the road to full recovery, the plaster cast would come off in a few weeks, and the coeliac disease was under control with a wheat-free diet. But he wasn't allowed to go home until he had spoken. It was Dr Rabjones's main concern, and a child psychiatrist from the Maudsley Hospital was on the case.

Then one morning it happened. And it was a cracker.

'Hello,' Dr Rabjones said to Angus. 'How are you today, little fella?'

'Not so bad,' Angus replied, in a broad Scots accent. 'How's yourself, wee man?'

I had never heard a man laugh with such uninhibited delight.

I'd been at the Belgrave for two months when Lisa was brought in with a swollen belly and severe abdominal pain.

A pretty girl with braided black hair, Lisa was twelve years old and the eldest of five daughters of African parents. Her father worked for British Rail while her mother stayed at home with the youngest children. Both parents were beside themselves with worry.

Suspecting our old friend appendicitis, the doctors

examined Lisa and performed the necessary tests, but when her white blood-cell count showed a normal result, and the pain was still present and considered too severe to be period pain, they ruled out the appendix and asked questions about pregnancy. Lisa's parents were now worried *and* horrified, and insisted there was no way their daughter could be pregnant. From that point on, the father steadfastly refused to leave Lisa's side.

When the pain showed no sign of easing, and was in fact escalating, it was suspected that Lisa had an ectopic pregnancy – that is, the embryo was developing in the fallopian tube instead of the uterus – and she was transferred to King's for further investigation and possible emergency surgery. I went with Lisa and her parents in the ambulance.

We were all thinking the worst and, thankfully, before Lisa was on the operating table, and before police could be summoned to subject the family to unthinkable questions, Lisa was examined by a consultant gynaecologist, who was in paroxysms of delight over his startling discovery.

Lisa wasn't pregnant. She had the rarest of things: a double uterus!

In normal female development, the uterus starts as two small tubes, which join to create one hollow tube that becomes a single uterus. In Lisa's case, her small tubes had never joined, so she had two uteri and also two vaginas, one closed and one with a cervix. The onset of puberty had triggered her symptoms, which the gynaecologist diagnosed as severe period pain with associated fluid retention that could be well managed in the future.

Surgery would not be necessary unless Lisa's pain

didn't subside, but as it finally disappeared after her first menstrual period commenced within three days, Lisa was sent home with a great story, drawings by the gynaecologist of her unique reproductive organs, strong medication to control future period pain, a follow-up appointment with the gynaecologist, who wasn't going to let anyone else look after his Rare Lisa, and the news that her diagnosis would not affect her having children in the future.

Even though everyone promised that Christmas at the Belgrave would be fun, with Santa and presents, I doubted that sick children and anxious parents trying to look happy would be a wild ride. Besides, I had three days off. I'd worked the last two Christmases and it was time I showed up for festivities at home. Richard and Esther were driving down from Newcastle, so the family would be together.

My friends – Jan, Kathy, Meredith, Miranda, Polly, Adele and Tilly – were either working or going home to their respective families, and Alistair was studying for his physician's exams and skiing in Austria. After Christmas, I would have another week at the Belgrave, then go straight to the operating theatres at King's, so there was no skiing for me.

Christmas at home was *almost* as I remembered from my childhood – the tree topped by the fat fairy in white lace, bowls of mandarins and walnuts, Jenny Dog wearing a red ribbon, snowball cocktails, a roaring fire, laughter, my mother's Dior perfume, dancing to Herb Alpert and the Tijuana Brass, turkey, dates, mince pies, a walk in the woods, the Queen's message and *The Great Escape* on television – but there was a major difference: my father's presence. I could count on one hand the number of Christmases he had spent at home during my lifetime. According to family legend, when Richard was three and our father had come home for Christmas, Herbie J was about to tuck into Christmas pudding when my brother had said, 'Those are my mother's spoons.' My father probably didn't need to be reminded of that.

There was talk of Richard and Esther's wedding in the coming August, and how it would be a simple register-office affair in Durham. So my father took a quantum leap and asked about Alistair and me.

'Worried I'm getting dusty on the shelf?' I teased him.

'Are you serious about each other?' he asked, looking a bit annoyed. I knew he wanted the full white-wedding catastrophe for me, an idea my mother and I abhorred.

'Sort of serious,' I told him. 'But I'm not even thinking about marriage until I'm thirty.'

'That's good,' my mother announced, sounding relieved. 'Still plenty of time for university and physics.'

I rolled my eyes at Mum. She narrowed hers at me. This was dangerous ground. I smiled at my father and wondered what my upbringing would have been like if it hadn't been entirely overseen by a free-thinking, strong-willed, capable female who didn't care what anyone thought, who believed sensitivity was a strength and failure an option, and who sprayed perfume on the pillows.

CHAPTER 14

Twenty-four Days
in A&E

King's College Hospital, London: Early 1973

ON THE COUNTDOWN of my final eight months as a student nurse, there was obvious urgency by the School of Nursing to accelerate areas of training that I hadn't experienced. In quick succession, I was scheduled to dip my toes into operating theatres, Casualty, Out-patients, William Bowman eye ward and Lonsdale male surgical ward, and all before a holiday with Alistair in Sardinia at the end of May.

'I'm not looking forward to the eye ward,' I told Jan and Kathy. 'I'm funny about eyes.'

The three of us were having drinks at the Fox on the Hill after my last shift at the Belgrave. It was the coldest winter day so far and our coats, scarves and gloves were piled high on a spare chair.

'If anything will make you throw in the towel, Maggie, it will be operating theatres,' Jan said, with confidence.

'Why is that?' I asked, a little testy as Jan had hit a

nerve. 'Don't you think I'm capable?' Secretly, you see, I was worried that I wasn't. 'Operating theatre' had an inexplicable grandness and mystique about it, as though it was where the real grown-ups worked. It was an alien world to student nurses: new sights, new words, new smells, new everything. Even British surgeons were not called 'Doctor' but were addressed as 'Mr'.

'Well?' I asked, when neither of my friends answered. I was tired and tetchy. We had all been to a nurses' ball at the Hilton Hotel in Park Lane the previous night and had grabbed a couple of hours' sleep before working all day. Screaming children had finished me off; my friends appeared far more resilient. I took a swig of lager; hair of the dog and all that.

Jan put down her drink and looked serious. 'More than capable, Maggie, but in theatre the doctors are demanding and the patients are unconscious.'

'So?'

'We're not doctors' assistants, Maggie,' Kathy interjected. 'We are patients' nurses.'

'Is this a roundabout way of telling me I don't take authority well?'

'You don't,' Jan said matter-of-factly, 'but there is no nurse–patient relationship in theatre. And you really will be a doctor's handmaiden.'

'So?' I said again. Then, realizing what a cow I was being, I apologized. 'Sorry, I'm not feeling myself today.'

'We noticed the improvement,' Kathy quipped, and I grinned at her.

God, I loved these girls.

*

180

Of all the operating theatres at King's – orthopaedic, general surgery, colorectal, ENT, and so on – I was sent to eye theatre. Just dandy.

I was, however, relieved to learn that Dr Wolfbane was busy knocking people out at another London hospital. His presence and my fear that I wasn't going to manage well in theatres were my main concerns.

But now there was a bigger issue. Eyes! And if, like me, you are uncomfortable in that area of anatomy, assisting at an enucleation (removal of a cancerous eye) is not the best idea. Being thrown in at the deep end does not force the squeamishness out of you.

To be honest, I couldn't see anything – the patient was swathed in acres of green drapes, and the surgeons and scrub nurses were blocking my view. It was the idea of what was happening that undid me.

Tasked with being a 'runner', it was my job to fetch and deliver things, and I calmed myself by breathing in through my nose and out through my mouth. This worked a treat until there was an almighty crash as I pitched head first into a trolley laden with used instruments. It is still the only time in my life I have fainted.

I lasted one day in eye theatre. Well, four hours if we are being picky. I was swiftly transferred to orthopaedic theatre, where strong men with saws and drills did wondrous things with bone and metal. It was carpentry on a grand scale. To Crosby, Stills and Nash.

Understandably, the surgeons couldn't be bothered with a student nurse fainting or passing the wrong clamps, so I counted used instruments and swabs and noted the numbers on a board. After the operation, I counted everything again to ensure no swabs or instruments had been left inside the patient. In between counting, I picked things up off the floor, answered the phone, held things, poured things and assisted the anaesthetist.

Night duty in theatre was markedly different from night-nursing in the lonely, ethereal lamplight of a darkened ward. For a start, all the lights were on, and it didn't matter how much noise we made. The workload was erratic: either nothing was happening and we drank coffee and cleaned instruments, or it was action stations as emergency cases were brought in one after another. Strangulated hernias, foreign bodies in throats, burst appendix, ruptured spleens from fist fights, major trauma from car accidents and stabbings, mauled arms and legs from a dog attack, cerebral bleeds, bones sticking out of legs: an endless list of calamity and misfortune.

If you didn't know what you were doing in an operating theatre, and I didn't, you were sensibly kept as far away as possible from an emergency operation. At such times my job, if I wasn't the runner, was to make coffee for the surgeons who were called from their beds, and to look after anxious relatives pacing the corridor outside. This night-time pacing was where I witnessed two of the most powerful human emotions: fear and hope.

King's was famous for the liver unit established by Professor Roger Williams in the sixties. A highlight of my night-duty theatre experience was being sent to another operating theatre where I was told a rare liver transplant was in progress. Standing at the back, it was impossible to see anything as some very tall people had also been invited, but I was there, jumping up and down for a glimpse, like a Jack Russell terrier trying to see out of a window. King's had the world's first specialist liver intensive-care unit for adults and today performs the most liver transplants in Europe. Sterling stuff for me, in the early days of liver transplants, to have almost seen the top of a surgeon's head.

Jan and Kathy were right about my disliking theatre. There wasn't a single day when I felt comfortable. For me, nursing was caring about patients, and caring for them. In theatre, patients were dehumanized on the operating table, and there was, as Jan had said, an impersonal nature to the nurse–patient relationship.

I fared better in the recovery room, where patients had a face and a voice, albeit groaning and retching when they came round from the anaesthetic. Recovery was a dangerous time for patients: they required constant observation and assessment. As a kipper, I was often alone looking after patients in recovery. Alone and, to be truthful, scared stiff.

Jan and Kathy were right about something else as well. I wasn't thrilled by the doctor–nurse relationship in theatre. It was far too master–slave for me. I could see no reason why a nurse was required to pass instruments to a surgeon. To me, it seemed an awful waste of a lot of nursing knowledge. Jan and Kathy both pretended to be surprised when I told them what I thought. And, to their credit, they resisted saying, 'We told you so.'

I had only three days left in theatre when I had the misfortune to work with Sister Tamora, an Irish theatre sister in her early thirties. She was, I'm fairly sure, a psychopath. Sweetness and light to doctors, Tamora was shamelessly cruel to junior nurses and medical students. I had seen her humiliate a female medical student and watched a staff nurse flee in tears after a confrontation with her.

It was my turn.

A hip replacement was in progress when the drama unfolded. Sister Tamora instructed me to pour normal saline into the kidney dish she was holding. I poured the liquid as requested but, with a quick flick of the wrist, Tamora shook the kidney dish towards me so that fluid spilled over my legs and shoes. A malevolent look enveloping her face, she threw the kidney dish on the floor. It hit the ground with a startling clang.

'How dare you throw things?' she shouted. 'Pick that up! Now!'

I was shocked and speechless. Clearly the woman was mad. I looked around. Had anyone seen? The surgeons and nurses were looking at us, but no one said anything.

Cautiously I picked up the kidney dish. The tirade that followed was indescribable. Having an attentive audience, Sister Tamora accused me of wasting hospital property and endangering a patient's life by causing a disturbance during an operation, and with relish she told me I was a dumb blonde who should be working at Woolworths.

During this foul invective, I stared at the fluid left in the bottle I was holding as if it were the most fascinating liquid on the planet. Eventually, in an almost involuntary action, I raised my arm and poured the remaining liquid over Tamora's head. Then I walked out. Straight to Sister Caroline's office. Still holding the bottle.

Oh, my goodness, what had I done? Surely this was the end of my career. Would Sister Caroline understand? Would anyone understand?

Sister Caroline did not question my teary explanation. Instead she left me shaking in her office and went to the operating theatre while I awaited her return, sick with worry. When she came back, her expression was serious. A surgeon and staff nurse had supported my story. I was reprimanded for responding to the sister's behaviour instead of reporting it, and, after writing my statement, I was sent home for dry shoes and stockings.

The next day, I was moved to Casualty at King's, where a staff nurse informed me that Sister Tamora had applied for a senior theatre position at another London hospital, and word was that she was being given a fantastic reference to make sure she got the job. This turn of events bothered me greatly. Not only had Tamora emerged unscathed, but she had probably secured a promotion and would carry on verbally harming people without redress.

In early 1973, Londoners were mindful that the Provisional IRA were expanding their bombing campaign in mainland Britain. In March, they planted four bombs in the capital. Two were defused and two exploded, one near the Old Bailey and the other in Whitehall.

On full alert, pedestrians avoided rubbish bins on pavements, cinema-goers checked under seats, Irish colleagues stopped speaking in public for fear of abuse, and people walked the length of Oxford Street rather than take the tube or a bus. And all hospitals were preparing for the worst.

This was a time when ambulances were white, nurses dressed in full regalia, and we called the Accident and

Emergency Department at King's College Hospital 'Casualty' or 'Cas'. It was fast-paced, bright and noisy, and everything ran on coffee and adrenalin. I loved it.

Unlike my experience in operating theatres, where nearly everything was unfamiliar, I was quite confident working in Casualty. In spite of six months' nursing on geriatric wards, I had already encountered many of the illnesses and accidents that I would come across in Cas, and I was also familiar with many emergency procedures.

Within Cas, there was a central waiting area packed with chairs on which sat the walking wounded – unless football was on television at home, in which case the waiting area was practically empty. During busy times, everybody complained about the long wait to be seen, except homeless men, who enjoyed the warmth and hot drinks we provided.

Along the side of the waiting area were individual rooms where doctors and nurses treated patients who needed to lie down. One room had two doors, one of which led to the outside of the building. It was there that, after a wash and a hot meal, we settled the homeless men for a nap in the hope that, when they woke up, they would open the outside door and disappear down to Camberwell Green and the homeless shelter. I lost count of the number of times I disinfected that room and replaced the blankets. Staff never grumbled about the homeless. After all, this was King's College Hospital. Come one, come all.

At the far end of the waiting area, behind a screen wall, doctors sat at desks and assessed ambulant patients: broken arms, twisted ankles, high fevers, dog bites, suspected TB, head lice, minor burns, hand lacerations – basically any injury or infection you could stagger in with.

After assessing these patients, the doctors wrote instructions for nurses on a chart. Treatment could be anything: strapping, bandaging, dressing wounds, organizing tests, cleaning wounds ready for suturing, giving tetanus shots, or admitting a patient to a main ward or to the small upstairs observation ward where patients (usually those who had received a bang on the head) were observed closely for twenty-four hours.

Time wasters – particularly drug addicts who feigned the intense pain of kidney stones in the hope of scoring pethidine – were offered help for their addiction, but they inevitably refused. If the addict was insistent that they be given drugs, or was abusive to the medical staff, it was not uncommon to see TTFO (tell to eff off) or GATKITT (give a therapeutic kick in the testicles) or STTTOL (straight to the Tower of London) written on our nursing instructions. These patients could become violent when refused drugs, and I'm sure our elaborate and authoritative nursing uniforms protected us. At times, the outfit could garner almost reverential respect from patients.

Around the corner from the waiting area, to the left of the doors at the ambulance entrance, was an emergency room. This was for dangerously ill patients who were brought in by ambulance. It was in that room that I helped pump out the stomachs of desperate overdose victims, removed a ball bearing from a hysterical child's nose, and watched a doctor cut open a young man's chest and massage the failing heart with his hand as tears rolled down his cheeks. I saw people die in that room, their relatives outside the door falling to the floor in grief. The worst was a RTA (road traffic accident) involving five teenagers, all horribly damaged, and some dead before morning. Sometimes, I can still see the mothers.

Notably, there were few re-admissions to Casualty of patients who had recently been discharged from hospital. This was, I think, mainly because people stayed in hospital longer back then – often, incredibly, until they were completely better!

The red phone that warned of an incoming serious case was in the main Casualty area. When it rang, the nearest person answered it, and everyone stopped and waited for instructions. 'Two minutes, two men, crush injuries from a building site!' someone shouted. Our adrenalin pumped as the team gathered in the emergency room to receive the injured patients, the wailing sirens coming closer . . .

For me, the best thing about Cas was renewing my friendship with Bernice, a student nurse in the set above me. A lovely north-country girl with the sandy complexion and hair of a Nordic blonde, Bernice had a gentle, easy manner and a winning smile, and we had worked together before and become good friends.

I enjoyed my time on Cas. I learned that misfortune can strike us at any time, and that a simple mistake may have life-changing consequences. And, forty-five years later, watching the British documentary *24 Hours in A&E*, it was immediately apparent to me that the same respectful King's rules that applied in my day are still in force.

Don't judge. Just care.

It's a mantra to live by.

*

Twenty-four Days in A&E

Outpatients' department kept regular hours, nine to five, Monday to Friday, and it was a stroll in the park compared with theatre and Cas. I worked in the fracture clinic, strapping broken fingers and sprained wrists, reapplying bandages and splints, removing sutures and teaching people how to fold and wear a sling, and the correct way to use crutches. By the end of my Outpatients' placement, I was ready to bandage for England at the Commonwealth Games.

Without pausing for breath, I moved on to William Bowman eye ward, which heralded an intense two-week period of avoiding anything to do with eyes. Fortunately, Willy Bowman was a modern ward in the new block that allowed a nurse to walk around corners carrying things and looking busy when she wasn't. There were many rooms to disappear into, and I spent a lot of time searching for an imaginary person for whom there was an imaginary phone call.

Next stop: Lonsdale, the male surgical ward at King's. Best news: the ward sister, Sister Annabelle, was an absolute honey. A large Nightingale ward, Lonsdale had a high patient turnover and a broad range of surgical nursing to learn. It was the male equivalent of the female surgical ward, Pantia Ralli, and with almost the same body parts – heart, bowel, lungs, pancreas, stomach and spleen – although not so many gall bladders.

Sister Annabelle steered a steady ship, and the ward was a busy and happy work environment. Annabelle was young and pretty, with a charming smile, and word was that if a nurse worked hard on Lonsdale, it would prove to be an exceptional learning period. I quickly found this to be true.

Unless there were complications during surgery, cardiac patients returned to the ward for post-operative care. A highlight for me was specialling a cardiac patient who had a modern pacemaker implanted in his chest to regulate his heartbeat. This was a year or so before lithium batteries were used, and patients remained in hospital for several days to ensure everything was working properly.

Back then, rest was considered paramount for recovery, and in addition to an enforced afternoon rest on many wards, visiting hours were limited to a set time, usually an hour, unless of course the patient was gravely ill. This restriction also allowed for more patient privacy on the Nightingale wards, where curtains around each bed were not always enough.

No experience, good or bad, is ever wasted, and I scored excellent Brownie points from Sister Annabelle when I displayed an encyclopaedic knowledge on colostomy care following a patient's bowel resection. I didn't think it necessary to mention that one of my childhood friends had had a colostomy and, because he was a typical kid, we all knew how a colostomy worked, as well as what you could do with the doings in the bag.

Times were changing for the better. Sister Annabelle called me Nurse Johnson on the ward and Maggie when we were in the clinical room or office. Previously, I had always been referred to by ward sisters as 'Johnson' and was rarely afforded the courtesy of 'Nurse Johnson'.

The patients were another matter. While they, the horizontal ones, knew the first names of every vertical angel, when they needed us urgently they would simply yell 'Nurse, quickly!' to which I and any other nurse in the vicinity would respond at a gallop. On Lonsdale, Nurse Quickly was shouted loud and often.

For a couple of days, we had a male agency staff nurse on Lonsdale. It was good to welcome him on board and wonderful to have male input into nursing care on the ward.

I considered it a great shame that there were no male student nurses in my set. I was a firm believer that male nurses would finally rid nursing of its women's-work image, and of the nonsensical 'calling' and 'vocation' labels. Women could demand reviews and lobby the government about better pay until the cows came home, but I was convinced that we would never attain decent working conditions, proper professional career paths and appropriate remuneration until many more male nurses started rolling off the assembly line.

My experiences working with Brad Hutchins on Fisk and Cheere had been overwhelmingly positive. I had teased Brad relentlessly that he would be called Mister Sister when he was promoted to ward sister, but male sisters were called 'charge nurses' – an appropriate name that defined the position, gave it a masculine twist and removed feminine and religious connotations.

Towards the end of my time on Lonsdale, a machine that I had not seen before appeared on the ward. About the size of a milk crate, it was called a computer, and it was on trial. Neither nurses nor doctors were allowed to touch the computer, so we touched it every time we walked past.

The computer's handler was a small, fox-faced woman in a white coat, and we all thought she was a doctor. 'Computers are the way of the future,' she said confidently. 'One day, they will replace nurses.'

That statement secured her destruction.

'You've been watching too much *Dr Who*,' a staff nurse told her and taped an 'Out of Sugar' sign on the computer while Dr Fox-face was at lunch.

Someone else (okay, that was me) stuck a label on the back that said 'Made by trolls in Middelfart, Denmark'. And the night nurses wrapped it in bandages.

Poor Dr Fox-face. She wasn't having a good time. We weren't impressed by her or her computer. She tutted and shook her head and fussed over the machine, but it didn't save a single life all week.

It was taken away in the night and we didn't see it or Dr Fox-face again.

You could tell there was no future in that sort of thing.

Life was busy, with much to look forward to: Richard and Esther's wedding in August, and a few days after that my parents' wedding anniversary and my twenty-first birthday. I was due to start my three-month obstetrics course, so I would need to set aside time to study for the obstetrics exam in mid-September and my state nursing finals on 1 October, but I wasn't going to let anything mar the rest of the summer, or my enjoyment of family celebrations.

As it turned out, I didn't have to worry about study wrecking things. There was a far more sinister script developing.

CHAPTER 15

Every Silver Lining Has
a Dark Cloud

*King's College Hospital, London: Summer, Autumn and
Early Winter, 1973*

OUR THREE MONTHS' obstetrics training took place that
summer. At King's, we rotated through ante-natal and
post-natal clinics, the community midwives, the
labour ward, the maternity ward, the nursery, where
labelled newborns slept, and the milk room, where we
made feeds for babies not on breast milk.

Since 1970, there had been rapid changes in
maternity care. Home deliveries, medically-induced
labour, and Caesarean sections were becoming more
common, as were episiotomies, which had previously
been viewed as emergency intervention. The development
of ultrasound also allowed mothers and babies who
were considered 'at risk' to be monitored, but the
practice was far from routine.

On the labour ward, I was introduced to one of the
most sobering sights I have ever seen. A young African
woman was in labour with her first child, but she had

193

undergone female circumcision, or female genital mutilation as it is also known. Her clitoris and most of her labia had gone, leaving an opening rigid with scar tissue. There was no skin left to stretch to allow the baby to leave the birth canal. If the baby survived the delivery, the mother risked being ripped to shreds, massive blood loss or a fistula forming into her bowel. A Caesarean section was performed and they both survived. I never saw such a thing again. It would be 1979 before the World Health Organization recommended that female circumcision should cease. Banned by many countries, it still happens as a cultural practice in parts of Africa, Asia and the Middle East.

Although the numbers were decreasing, many women were still giving birth at home, assisted by a midwife. And, in London, help at a major hospital was never far away. These mothers and babies were looked after by a mix of the National Health Service, the local doctor and the local council (which then managed most community health services).

As part of the community component of my obstetrics training, I was sent to facilitate ante-natal classes in a community hall on a run-down housing estate in South London. It was a desolate, soulless place, with a lot of brickwork, cracked concrete, boarded-up windows and mean-looking boys on bicycles.

At about the same time, on a similar housing estate, Alistair was visiting a patient while working as a GP locum. He was sitting in the driver's seat of his Triumph Stag, with the top down and reading medical notes, when the paper he was holding blew on to the floor on the passenger side. He leaned over to retrieve it and heard a shot. A bullet hit the back of the driver's seat, missing him by a millisecond. Alistair drove out of there like the devil was chasing him. It's a story that gives an idea of what conditions were like on some housing estates back then – it certainly wasn't the Cotswolds.

On my first day, ten mothers-to-be awaited me in a hall that smelt of vomit and urine. The chairs had disappeared and the women were sitting around on the floor, comparing tattoos and discussing weekend visits to their menfolk in prison.

I politely said good morning and walked to the front, where I stuck a chart of a baby coming down a birth canal on the wall. No one took the slightest bit of notice of me, not even when I said *vagina* very loudly.

On day two, I asked one of the women to put out her cigarette. Sneering, she threw some verbal abuse my way, which I took to be a positive step. At least we were communicating, but not enough for the midwife overseeing my community placement. Declaring that I had failed birth classes, she moved me elsewhere. And that was how I found myself on a rubber mat taking the exercise clinic for twenty heavily pregnant ladies.

These women hated me even more than the birth-class group, and because I wouldn't let them smoke while doing exercises, I was considered evil.

'Swing those legs,' I called.

'Oh, sod off,' they yelled, and flicked cigarette ash on the floor.

I was saved from a second teaching failure by a large West Indian woman called Veronica, who was expecting her ninth child, so she needed my help – a lot. She respectfully called me 'Nurse', and smiled and told me that her husband had named their eight children after British prime ministers. This, she said, had caused a problem with her two daughters, who were eventually named Clementine after Clement Attlee and Charlene after Charles Grey.

My, could Veronica laugh. Her whole body shook and she folded her arms under her large breasts and shook those too. Tears rolled down her face, and she would fall to the floor and laugh and laugh as she slammed the floor with her fists. I became hostage to Veronica's good humour and directed my words and demonstrations towards her.

One day, I positioned the mothers on their hands and knees and taught them to swing their behinds from side to side and turn their heads at the same time, an exercise designed to strengthen the spine during pregnancy.

'Come on, Veronica,' I chirped, 'bend that lovely bottom to the side and turn that pretty head.'

'Oh dear,' Veronica complained wistfully, 'it's doing this that got me here in the first place.'

We all collapsed with laughter. And we laughed and cried and rolled around on the floor, and, like Veronica, slammed the linoleum with our fists.

This was the scene that greeted the midwife overseeing my community placement.

'May I see you outside?' she said.

Past caring if I was in trouble or not, I jumped up and wiped my eyes with a towel. As I left the room, I remarked flippantly over my shoulder, 'Take a rest, girls.' Personally speaking, it was a very professional moment.

'I must say,' the midwife effused, as she jumped aside when a youth on a bicycle with a car radio under his arm sped between us, 'you have struck a chord with these mothers that no one else has managed. I will make reference to it in my report.'

'Thank you,' I said, smiling like a fool. I tried not to look proud but I had succeeded where others had failed. I was going to receive a good report. Now all I had to do was pass the obstetrics exam.

A beam of sunlight broke through a cloud and shone on a row of determined daisies that had grown through a crack in the concrete. For a few seconds, the housing estate almost looked pretty.

The end of summer would sound the bell for the second life-changing tragedy to hit the Johnson family.

My mother had always been unnecessarily frugal with herself, cutting her own hair, making her own clothes and riding a bicycle everywhere instead of using the car. I could never figure out if it was a hangover from the war years or if she was punishing herself for something. Finally I learned that it had always been her intention to save enough money for my father to retire early from the Merchant Navy, which he had done, and for them to share their remaining years together. A glorious, well-earned future lay ahead. They enjoyed it for less than a year.

On the day of Richard and Esther's wedding in Durham on 20 August 1973, my mother tripped at the reception, fell down and broke her hip. My brother was concerned. You don't break your hip from a fall like that, he said. Our mother was admitted to the Newcastle Royal Victoria Infirmary.

A few days later, on my parents' wedding anniversary and my twenty-first birthday, Richard told me that Mum, who was only forty-nine years old, had carcinomatosis – multiple cancers developing in many organs that had spread from a primary source – and she had, at most, three months to live. Like Mrs Barnes on the gynae ward at Dulwich Hospital, my mother had not felt well for a while but had delayed seeking help because of family commitments.

My parents returned to Hindhead and I left King's and our shared house to care for my mother. A short time later, one of her kidneys, a suspected primary source of the cancer, was removed at Guildford Hospital. It was a desperate move, but a hopeless one. Things were too far gone, and an ambulance brought my beautiful mother home for me to look after.

Somewhere in the nightmare, I went to London and sat my obstetrics exam, oral exams, my state nursing finals and something called a hospital exam. I don't remember any of it, but I know that I couldn't have managed anything without the support of my friends and Sister Caroline. I owe them more than I can say, especially Jan, Kathy and Bernice.

There were other concerns too. Having left King's, I had lost my income and was too proud to ask my father for financial help. When I first went home, I had applied to the government for the nursing carer's allowance that was available. I was told by an officious woman on the phone that a staff member would come to our house and visit my mother to assess my validity to claim. She sounded suspicious, as though I were staging an elaborate hoax.

In October 1973, Queen Elizabeth II officially opened Sydney Opera House in Australia. It was televised, and I sat beside my mother on her bed and held her hand as we watched the ceremony.

'Just look at that fancy building,' my mother managed

breathlessly, but she was staring out of the bedroom window. Her eyes were sunken and her dry mouth was making speech difficult. I popped a small, lime-flavoured ice cube that I had dipped in gin into her mouth.

I was spellbound by the sun shining down on the magnificent white roof of Sydney Opera House, the harbour awash with yachts and white caps, and the formidable backdrop of that most famous of coat-hangers, Sydney Harbour Bridge.

'Is the roof supposed to resemble sails or shells?' I asked Mum.

She focused on the television. 'It looks like shark fins to me.'

There was a howling gale blowing in Sydney, making it difficult to hear the Queen's speech – but, oh, the light, the people, the smiles . . . It was magical.

'Bloody awful hat,' Mum said, of the Queen's millinery effort.

Ignoring her, I announced with certainty, 'I'm going to live in Sydney one day.'

'I expect you will,' Mum said at length, and then she sighed again. 'You could work anywhere with your nursing qualification.' Gently, she squeezed my hand. 'If you pass the exam, which you will.'

'I will,' I said confidently, and squeezed her hand back. Would she live to find out?

'It's not for you, is it, a normal life?' she said wearily.

'What do you mean?'

'A white wedding, settling down, village life' – she took a big breath before continuing – 'children, a house with a garden, a husband with a proper job and a good income? You crave more excitement, don't you?'

I laughed. 'I suppose I do, but that's your fault. You didn't raise me to be mousewife material.'

When my mother didn't respond, I looked across at her. She had fallen asleep. Too many words; too much effort. Still holding her hand, I lay back on the pillow with my head beside hers and wept silently.

It seems like only a few years ago that my mother died. But I am now fifteen years older than she was at her death.

It was on the morning of her funeral that I learned I had passed my state finals and hospital exam and that I was a qualified state registered nurse. Somehow, I had also passed my obstetrics exam.

No one said well done. No one cared. Not even me.

I remember nothing of my mother's funeral. Except that *Marion Johnson* was engraved on her coffin.

The following morning, a woman from social services turned up to assess my situation for the carer's allowance. It was a while since I had applied. I told her to go away, but I think not in those words.

Richard and Esther returned to Newcastle, where they were both working, and Alistair, Jan, Kathy and Bernice rallied round me with support. Looking back, I see that I was emotionally and physically adrift for several months. I had lost my anchor and was tossing in turbulent seas over the responsibility of taking care of my bereft father, who was drunk on whisky and grief, and the pressing personal need to earn my own living.

Encouraged by friends, I went up to King's to see Sister Caroline and collect my certificates and badges. It transpired that I wouldn't be receiving anything until I had made up the time I had lost while caring for my mother, and from excess sick leave taken during my training. The excess leave was due to recurrences of illness following glandular fever, but I think it would have been overlooked had I not been sprung that time at the Tutankhamun exhibition. Somehow I had known that trickery would come back to bite me.

It seemed unfair, as Sister Caroline pointed out, but it was out of her hands. Having to make up the time, she said, was probably the best thing that could happen to me as it forced me to return to London, my friends and my work. She was kind and sympathetic, and generous with her praise for my care of my mother and passing the exams.

Jan, Kathy and Bernice were living in the downstairs half of a shared house in Beckwith Road, Herne Hill, and I moved in with them. Trying hard to ignore the fact that Kip was living upstairs with Roman and another student, Mark, I just got on with it, working and dividing my time between London and my father's house in Hindhead. My goal was to earn money quickly, as I didn't have a bean to my name, and make up the nursing time so I could collect my certificates and badges. Fed up with penury, I was looking forward to my first decent pay cheque as a qualified staff nurse.

I went home for the first Christmas after my mother's death to spend time with my father, brother and sister-in-law and, for us, the festive season was awash with harrowing grief. Fraught with loss, my father cooked a Christmas pudding that my mother had made in July and frozen, and when we were all too upset to eat it, he raged about betrayal and wasted food

CHAPTER 16

The Two Musketeers

Savoy Hotel, London: March 1974

'I DON'T BELIEVE it!' I shrieked.

Looking down at the sodden slip of paper in my hand, I swore angrily – colourful words that would have made my father blush. This was *not* how the much-anticipated opening of my first pay slip as a qualified state registered nurse was supposed to play out.

Having finished a late shift as a staff nurse at King's, I'd been so eager to celebrate finally achieving my goal that, rather than wait for a bus, I had sprinted home in the dark and the pouring rain to our shared house in Beckwith Road. And I'd been singing.

Dripping on to the threadbare carpet in the living room, I wondered if the paltry amount was a mistake. After all, I had made up the required time *and* worked as a staff nurse on the private patients' wing for a month.

'This is only a few quid more than I earned as a student,' I complained to Bernice. She was kneeling on the floor in front of the fire, ironing her staff nurse's bonnet.

'Here, let me see,' she said.

I passed her the pay slip and paced up and down.

'No, that's right,' Bernice said eventually. She had been a staff nurse on the private wing at King's for a while, but, incredibly, we had never discussed pay. I'd just assumed she was earning grown-up money. I mean, didn't everyone when they qualified at something?

'Chin up, Mags,' Bernice said encouragingly. 'I thought the idea of celebrating tonight was to make a significant memory of your new professional status, not blow our trumpets over the amount you were paid.'

Bernice was right. Money aside, grief and disappointment had been firing poisoned arrows at me broadside for six months and I desperately needed to mark my qualification with a pleasant memory to transcend the real one. There had been no excitement when I'd passed my finals – just endless days of ineffable sadness.

My head in the sand, I had foolishly anticipated a decent reward for years of study and hard physical work. I wasn't expecting piles of money – I wasn't that stupid – but somehow I hadn't drawn the connection between the years of national whining over poor nurses' pay and my own situation. I could almost hear my mother saying, *I told you so.*

Flopping on to the sofa, I had a fleeting vision of the future: an empty, colourless life of making do and doing without until I was found starving to death in a run-down old caravan on the edge of a cliff at an abandoned holiday park in Cornwall.

'Mags, you're soaked,' Bernice said, interrupting my thoughts. 'Go and change and we'll open the champagne. We'll make a good memory, you'll see.'

It burned me that my mother hadn't known I had passed my finals, and I was now aggrieved that she wasn't witnessing the pay slip. For sure, if there was a God, he was a mean-spirited, spiteful bastard not to let her have the final word.

Moving away from thoughts that triggered maudlin self-pity, I sought refuge in analysis of my most marvellous financial stupidity – anger at oneself is a much safer harbour than sorrow. 'How could I not know how much I'd be paid?' I remonstrated aloud with myself.

Screwing up the pay slip, I went to my room and changed before rejoining Bernice. It was just the two of us for champagne, as Jan was on night duty, Kathy was having dinner with her mother in the East End, and Alistair was on call on the other side of London.

Bernice opened the first of the two bottles of champagne I had bought.

'Congratulations!' she said, and we clinked glasses. The champers wasn't especially cold, because our fridge didn't do especially cold, but it tasted good to our pedestrian palates, and it made my nose tickle.

'Do you want the lads to join us?' Bernice asked.

We could hear Mark, Kip and Roman stomping about upstairs.

I shook my head. The truth was that living in the same house as my ex-boyfriend, Kip, was awkward for both of us and I tried to avoid him where possible. I knew that if he looked at me and smiled, I would be goose-meat.

'More for us, then,' Bernice said, grinning over her glass.

We made small-talk for a while, avoiding anything to do with work and pay, until Bernice said, 'You know, we all expect more money when we qualify. I did.'

I chewed this over and decided that Bernice was being kind. After all, kindness was her default position. But was I being too hard on myself? Maybe my blistering ignorance was because I was born in a time when it was considered bad form to discuss money.

In the interest of self-preservation, I did a mental gear shift, finally settling on an explanation that shared the blame nicely. I reasoned that for years everyone had been beguiled by the romantic paradigm that nursing was a vocation, and that this vocation was being amply rewarded by simply allowing a nurse to train and work as a nurse. Ergo, no grand remuneration from the state coffers was necessary.

Well, stuff that.

I shared my thoughts with Bernice.

'We should have taken industrial action in 'seventy-two,' Bernice said ruefully, 'with the other workers.'

I nodded. 'We should.'

The cork from the second bottle hit the ceiling and ricocheted off the television, and we toasted the Queen and Battersea Dogs Home. Then, with commendable dexterity, we used rulers, sticky tape and envelopes to make small placards that said WE WANT MORE MONEY and DOWN WITH THIS SORT OF THING.

Half an hour later, our stomachs sore from laughing, we penned our formal resignations from King's College Hospital.

'That'll . . . you know . . . sh-show 'em,' Bernice said and hiccuped loudly.

'Yesh,' I said, raising my glass. 'Teach the fooze to pay us pwoply.'

We'd made a good memory all right . . .

*

The Two Musketeers

Mid-morning, and still intent on our plan, Bernice and I caught the bus to King's. Two dangerous radicals, we assumed a defiant air as we marched into the hospital and handed in our resignations at the administration office.

It wasn't as satisfying as we had anticipated. Without looking at us, the secretary tossed our resignations into a pigeon hole behind her desk and resumed typing. No nursing officers threw themselves at our feet and begged us to stay. No one said goodbye and good luck. They didn't need to. It was the seventies and times had changed. There was a rearguard of girls leaving school to pursue a nursing career rather than jump straight into marriage.

Disappointed, we bought Mars bars for solace and scoffed them on the way home, unaware that we were not alone in taking a stand over our pay and conditions. Not by a long shot. But the year was still young and Bernice and I were ignorant of imminent national rumblings. We worked our notice and left the mother ship with our heads held rebelliously high.

Agreeing to spend our meagre severance pay wisely, we visited Regent's Park Zoo on Sunday, the Edvard Munch exhibition on Monday and the flicks in Leicester Square to see *The Way We Were* on Tuesday.

Emerging from the cinema into the gloomy grey afternoon, we walked through the city to the Savoy Hotel, where anyone who is anyone has afternoon tea.

Except we were not there for afternoon tea.

Flat broke, but culturally replete, we were attending an interview to become chambermaids.

Sitting high on a wide ribbon of land between the Strand and the Thames, the Savoy Hotel is a stately nineteenth-century icon overlooking Victoria Embankment Gardens and the river. It was, and still is, one of the most exclusive hotels on earth.

Built by the Gilbert and Sullivan impresario Richard D'Oyly Carte on proceeds from *The Mikado*, the guest list has always been a walk through an international *Who's Who*. Under the warm glow from its crystal chandeliers, Laurence Olivier wooed Vivien Leigh, and Princess Elizabeth first appeared in public with Prince Philip. Elsewhere in the hotel, Claude Monet painted the Thames from a balcony, Winston Churchill lunched with his cabinet, and Auguste Escoffier created Peach Melba and Melba Toast for the Australian soprano Dame Nellie Peach-Melba-Toast.

Was the Savoy Hotel, I asked Bernice, as we stood in Savoy Court and stared up at the iconic art-deco sign over the front entrance, ready for two lesser-known dames with just as much attitude as old Nellie?

'You'll have to go round the back,' the smartly uniformed doorman told us, with a twinkle in his eye. 'This entrance is for hotel guests.'

Surprised, I asked politely, 'How do you know we're not guests?'

He grinned broadly in response.

'Do you have any experience making beds?' Mrs Peters asked us. A study in servile black, the Savoy housekeeper had friendly eyes. She bore absolutely no resemblance to the skinny, hook-nosed harridan I had imagined.

'Oh, yes, lots,' I said, and Bernice nodded her agreement.

'Where?' Mrs Peters asked.

The Two Musketeers

Momentarily stumped, I could sense Bernice struggling not to laugh. We could probably make beds under general anaesthetic, but for fear of being thought overqualified we had agreed not to mention our nursing credentials.

'At home,' I said, after a long pause. 'I've made my bed for years.'

Mrs Peters chuckled. 'Both of you follow me,' she said cheerfully, and stood up.

After a few carpeted miles, Mrs Peters unlocked and opened a door into a beautifully furnished bedroom. Centre stage was the largest bed I had ever seen, and Mrs Peters demonstrated how to make a 'Savoy' bed. The bedding was exquisite: fine linen sheets hand-sewn by Irish leprechauns, pillows filled with the gossamer feathers of turtle doves, and blankets woven from the wings of cherubs – that sort of thing. I stroked the blanket while Mrs P showed us how to place a large fold in the top sheet at the foot of the bed, 'so that his lordship's feet are not crushed'.

'Your turn,' Mrs Peters said, as she pulled the bedding off the bed.

Not surprisingly, Bernice and I managed it easily, with precision-perfect corners.

'You're nurses, aren't you?' Mrs Peters said, grinning at us.

'Yes,' we said in unison. There seemed little point in denying it, but inwardly I sighed. One day, hopefully, someone would ask me if I was an artist or a journalist.

'That's good,' Mrs Peters said. 'I can trust you to work together on the same floor.'

Oh my, it sounded as though we already had jobs.

Our tasks, she explained, would be to make beds,

remove used linen and towels, clean the marble bathrooms, dust and polish the furniture and vacuum the floors. Glassware, lamps, mirrors and telephones would be cleaned by other staff. When a guest rang the bell, we were to knock on the door, wait to be invited in, then either respond to the request or alert the relevant staff member.

It sounded good to us.

'Any questions?' Mrs Peters asked.

'Yes,' Bernice said. 'How much will we earn?'

I blushed fire-engine red. Maybe subconsciously I did consider it bad form to discuss money.

The enquiry was readily answered: £18.22 a week before tax – roughly the amount we earned as qualified nurses. And with far less responsibility.

Two blondes dressed for a French farce, we started work at the Savoy on 4 March 1974.

Our friends thought we were nuts. Jan was a staff nurse at King's, Adele was ensconced in midwifery, Miranda and Polly were completing their health-visitor training, Kathy was working for an educational toy firm in the city, Meredith had returned to Canada and we had lost touch with Tilly, who had gone abroad with Klaus some time ago. All moving forward with their lives, their general reaction was that Bernice and I were moving backward with ours.

Mrs Peters allocated us to an upper floor of luxury suites that included the residence of the hotel's largest shareholder, Bridget D'Oyly Carte. And I mean that Miss D'Oyly Carte owned a sizeable chunk of the Savoy, which was built by her grandfather, not that she was a sizeable lady.

We were introduced to the butler, valets and floor waiters, and informed that Mrs Peters would cast an expert eye over our work, which she did for a couple of days and praised our thoroughness. Standards were high at the Savoy, and we kept with the programme, although it wasn't difficult. It was easy and pleasant polishing beautiful furniture and making beds in glorious surroundings. Scrubbing marble bathrooms that were never really dirty wasn't too taxing either.

Once a nurse, always a nurse, and no matter how hard Bernice and I tried, we couldn't un-nurse ourselves. Word quickly spread that we were state registered nurses and before long our new colleagues requested advice – not for themselves, you understand, but for a 'friend'. Our opinion was sought on bunions, chilblains, constipation, haemorrhoids, acne, boils, headaches, rashes, coughs, varicose veins, blocked ears and Aunt Maureen's embarrassing leak, and although we knew the answers, we were aware of professional limitations and recommended further advice be sought from a doctor. It was amazing, really. Even from afar, we were keeping the National Health Service in business.

Which brings me to Iris, a chambermaid in her sixties from whom strange noises were coming as she and I made a bed together. Iris had a friend, she said, who'd had a mastectomy and was wearing a plastic bag filled with birdseed in her empty bra cup to balance things up.

Touched by the poor woman's plight, and purposely avoiding looking at her in case she thought I was examining her chest, I said gently, 'Iris, you must tell your friend there are special places where you . . . I mean she . . . can be fitted with a proper artificial breast for the bra. I'll find some phone numbers for you . . . err . . . to give to her.'

Iris nodded, then turned away and busily plumped pillows.

Me too.

The frenetic bell-ringing set my heart pounding. I rushed to see which hotel room it was coming from.

A hospital nurse first and a chambermaid second, I automatically prepared myself to deal with a heart attack, choking or a severed artery.

Ring, ring, ring, ring, ring, ring. The bell clamoured on.

It was coming from the suite where the American model and actress Ann Turkel was staying. Hastily I walked along the hallway and banged on the door. 'Miss Turkel,' I called anxiously. 'Is everything all right?'

The door flew open and an alarmingly drunk Richard Harris, glass in hand, swayed in the doorway. You couldn't mistake him. A marvellous Irish actor, his performance was so good that I really believed he was totally hammered.

Hearing laughter in the background, I relaxed a little, but I was annoyed by my alarmist response to what had apparently been a highly amusing Irish method of summoning a servant girl. Taking a deep breath, I curtseyed and chanted, 'You rang, you rang, you rang, you rang, you rang, you rang . . .'

Momentarily stunned, Richard Harris quickly recovered and barked, 'More ice!' Then he slammed the door.

Naturally, I alerted the butler to the life-threatening

ice shortage in the Harris suite. It was, after all, the Savoy, and standards had to be maintained.

The following morning, while making up the Harris suite, retaliatory options crossed my mind. I thought about writing 'This book belongs to Ann R. Sole' on the inside cover of the novel *Strumpet City* that Harris was reading. I contemplated taking his rugby shirt out of the bidet where he had left it and putting it in the toilet instead. I pondered making an apple-pie bed. But I did nothing at all because Miss Turkel was such a peach.

I later learned that Richard Harris was reported to have been a vocal supporter of the Provisional IRA during the time that Bernice and I worked at the Savoy. Trust me, if I had known that at the time, I would have gone for the apple-pie bed.

Our employment at the Savoy coincided with the premiere in London of *The Three Musketeers*, the star-studded film of the Alexandre Dumas swashbuckling novel of the same name. Several of the stars were staying at the Savoy, and Geraldine Chaplin and Raquel Welch had suites on our floor. I didn't meet Miss Chaplin, but I did have the pleasure of attending to the needs of the charming and extraordinarily lovely Miss Welch.

My unpleasant cleaning experience on Dickens had cast a long shadow, and the stark contrast between wiping a commode at St Giles and polishing an antique chair at the Savoy (while Miss Welch removed the creases from an evening gown by holding it over a steaming kettle) did not escape me. While I abhorred the former and enjoyed the latter, I had nevertheless applied the same high standards to both. But cleaning inanimate objects, wherever they are, lacks any emotional response, and it was slowly dawning on me that emotional response was the prize I sought. Let's face it, no chair ever says, 'Thank you.'

Apart from sharing domestic chores with Miss Welch, there were other compensations at the Savoy, and one of them was meeting the hotel's most illustrious resident, Bridget D'Oyly Carte. A handsome woman in her sixties, Miss Bridget had warm, intelligent eyes, an aristocratic bearing and a cultured voice that was a little gravelly from smoking. An intensely private person, she nevertheless chatted up a storm while I cleaned her apartment at the Savoy. My work in her rooms always took longer than it should have, but I knew I was safe from reprimand. Along with heading the D'Oyly Carte Opera Company and controlling the rights to Gilbert and Sullivan, Miss Bridget was vice chairman of the Savoy, so who was going to tell me off?

Miss Bridget's illustrious CV belied a strong social conscience, which became apparent as we talked. In her younger days, she had worked for several years in child welfare, and we discussed rickets and other diseases of poverty that she hoped we had seen the back of. I know she was quietly amused that Bernice and I had taken such a drastic stand against our profession, and from the way she spoke I sensed she rather admired our nursing qualifications, which offered such a rewarding career. A kind and thoughtful lady, she generously gave me free theatre tickets when she discovered I liked opera and musical theatre, and I appreciated the warmth and interest she showed in a lowly chambermaid. She was, as they say, quite a dame.

The Two Musketeers

There was no doubt that respect for our nursing qualifications had secured Bernice and me our positions at the Savoy, and allowed the housekeeper to trust us to work together. Nursing appeared to be a passport to a range of possible jobs, although none of them well paid. We would never starve, but we would never have the bother of a country estate either.

Bernice and I worked as chambermaids at the Savoy for a month, and we both missed nursing. A lot. We missed the patients, the sense of purpose, the mental stimulation, the camaraderie on the wards, and the satisfaction that comes with well-managed responsibility.

Thanking Mrs Peters for our time at the Savoy, Bernice returned to King's, where she was welcomed back as a staff nurse on the private patient wing. I bought two powder-blue, knee-length nurse's uniform dresses with white collars, short sleeves and big hip pockets, and joined a nursing agency, the British Nursing Association (BNA).

The BNA paid higher wages than the National Health Service, and as a state registered nurse I could easily secure work in London at short notice. I was paid only for the days I worked, but I needed flexibility so that I could hoof off to Hindhead and spend time with my father, who wasn't coping well and whose drinking binges were escalating.

By late April, it was impossible to miss the national rumblings and threats of strike action by nurses for more pay. I was pleased that Bernice and I had already taken a stand in a small way, even though, as we had discovered to our surprise at the Savoy, money was not the ultimate prize.

CHAPTER 17

Everybody Out!

Agency Nursing, London: Spring and Summer 1974

'EVERYBODY OUT!' WAS a famous catchphrase of the sixties British comedy series *The Rag Trade*, which was set in a clothing factory. At the slightest hint of workplace injustice, the militant shop steward blew her whistle and shouted, 'Everybody out!' at which workers downed tools and viewers fell about laughing.

Who knew that the same catchphrase could have a more sinister meaning, and that nobody would be laughing on that cold spring morning in 1974 when I and hundreds of other commuters responded urgently to a bomb scare at a London tube station?

Until then I had been alert to recent Provisional IRA bombings in London, but I hadn't really been alarmed. Had I inherited the stoic, gritty resolve peculiar to the British? Or was my lacklustre concern a consequence of the ignorance, insouciance and invincibility of youth? Whatever, my attitude changed the day I was evacuated from that tube station. And even though the bomb scare turned out to be a hoax, for me the threat was suddenly real, and from that point on I was alert *and* alarmed.

Since last Christmas, the Provisional IRA had

already detonated bombs at Madame Tussaud's and the Boat Show in Earl's Court, and major London hospitals were now on standby with bomb protocols for emergency evacuation and receiving large numbers of casualties. Nurses and doctors were encouraged, in the event of a catastrophic attack in the capital, to carry identification when off duty and attend their nearest hospital to assist where needed.

Where possible, my friends and I made changes to our daily lives in order to avoid places that might be potential targets – transport hubs and London landmarks – and if we had a dinner date, we dined at out of the way restaurants in Battersea and Lewisham, which we felt were safer than central London.

Unfortunately for me, use of transport hubs was unavoidable, as I regularly ran the gauntlet of Waterloo station to catch the train home to visit my father. Still dealing with my own grief, I was having trouble coping with my father's escalation in drinking and his resultant distressing phone calls asking if I had seen my mother as she hadn't come home.

Often in tears, I was smoking heavily and my shoulders were sagging under the burden of responsibility. And for too long that responsibility was all mine, as my brother Richard was busy and couldn't easily get away from his hospital to help. Thankfully, my ever practical and thoughtful Aunt Joan, whom I adored, realized I was struggling and pitched in, cooking meals and curbing my father's drinking – a situation for which I was truly appreciative and, I later discovered, so was he!

Along with my friends and family, work was my salvation. There was oodles of agency nursing to choose from across London – and at times an extremely long walk home on days when I had a 'gut feeling' that today was the day something bad was going to happen on the tube.

Agency nursing could also be a trap-laden path, propelling me into situations where I had little experience but thought I would be okay. The idea of working on an acute infectious-diseases ward and bringing joy to lonely souls in isolation appealed to me but, never having nursed patients infected by diseases that could kill you, the reality scared the pants off me when I had to face it. After the second nightmare, when I dreamed I succumbed to enteric fever and the name Typhoid Maggie was stuck on the bed, I requested a transfer to a general ward.

Another time, I put my foot down at a hospital where I was allocated to a surgical ward *plus* the crash team. This was the small team of doctors and nurses who, in addition to their regular workload, responded to cardiac arrests within the hospital. Plainly it was dangerous to have an agency staff nurse unfamiliar with the hospital layout on the crash team. I said as much to the sister in charge and surprised myself by refusing to do it.

The sister went ramrod stiff, like an Easter Island statue. Slowly, like so many sisters before her, she turned puce. Unlike me, she was not impressed by my assertiveness, and I was sent to a geriatric ward to think about my behaviour. And that was the beauty of agency nursing: I didn't have to do something I considered wrong, or work on a ward I didn't like. The next day I could be sent somewhere else. It was pick and choose on a grand scale, and for the first time in my life I was earning decent money and saving easily.

Agency nursing taught me to have confidence in my own abilities and opinions. And it allowed me, with the support of the agency, safely to question entrenched attitudes and practices that I considered to be wrong. These included the expectation of many hospitals that agency nurses would work overtime without being paid for it, and the unkind practice I found at one hospital of waking sedated patients at 5 a.m. in order to bath everyone and have them looking spiffy for the doctor's early round.

Since my mother's death, I had also noticed a marked elevation in my empathy for patients' relatives. The new me took time to ask how they were, if there was anything they needed to know, whether they would like a cup of tea or to see Sister or the doctor. It wasn't that I hadn't cared about them before, but more that I hadn't actually considered them as part of the hospital equation. Often I'd thought of them as simply in the way. My focus was on the patient in a rather proprietary manner, but having been on the other side of the fence, I now understood what relatives and friends were experiencing – the angst, the sleepless nights, the endless phone calls to others – and that everything, all their wishes, was packaged in hope.

Agency nursing also revealed to me that all teaching hospitals functioned much like King's, which was a surprise. There was a healthy rivalry between the medical and nursing schools at the oldest London teaching hospitals – St Thomas' Hospital (nicknamed Tommy's), King's College Hospital (King's or KCH), St George's Hospital (George's), St Bartholomew's Hospital (Barts), Guy's Hospital, University College Hospital (UCH) and Westminster Hospital – and we all knew stories that made other hospitals sound like an East End knacker's yard and our own like a cross between Mary

Poppins's parlour and NASA. A standing joke among students was to tease others that you had 'Do not take me to [insert name of rival hospital here]' tattooed on your chest in case you were ever in an accident.

Medics generally thrashed out their competition on the rugby field, while most of us nurses maintained the belief, with quiet dignity and polished badges, that our own teaching hospital was the best. Proud as peacocks in our ridiculous bonnets, we were loyal to a fault.

By the end of June 1974, the phrase 'Everybody out!' was expanding its target audience into the Mediterranean. Cordialities between Greece and Turkey were beyond strained, and the two countries were on the brink of war. So, naturally, I was with Kathy and Bernice on a Greek island, slap bang off the coast of Turkey. Now I could worry about being blown to smithereens outside England as well as within it.

On our return to London, we learned that while we were away the Provisional IRA had detonated a bomb at the Houses of Parliament. Then, in mid-July, when I was working at Westminster Hospital, they detonated another bomb at the Tower of London, killing one person and causing many dreadful injuries.

Nowhere felt safe.

After Greece, I settled back into agency nursing in London and was soon working with Bernice again on the private patient wing at King's. Jan was a staff nurse on Lonsdale at King's, Kathy was planning to move back to Birmingham and marry Dave, and Alistair was preparing to fly to Canada for a six-week medical locum.

On the private wing, we cared for a range of medical

and surgical cases, and our patients numbered a few celebrities, high-profile businessmen, wealthy Arabs and soldiers injured in a foreign war. It was an interesting mix, which could attract unwelcome attention, and we all knew the evacuation procedure if there was a bomb threat.

At the time, we were caring for a well-known American actress, and she might be pleased to know that because she was such a brave, sweet and gentle lady, a few of us decided we would carry her out first if the order ever came to evacuate.

Second on our evacuation list was the lead guitarist from the biggest rock band in the world at the time. And the large stuffed penguin that was sitting on his bedside locker. He was a model patient, and the only thing he smashed was the image that rock stars were zonked-out, self-centred lunatics. He was the charming boy next door, except with a lot of hair. He gave each of the nurses an LP signed by all the band members, which I boasted about and played incessantly until it went west when I left it on the record player and the whole stereo was pinched. Maybe I had played it *too* often.

I also looked after a property developer whom I shall call Harry because that was his name. Harry was much in the news for allowing squatters to inhabit a large empty building of his in central London. Everyone – reporters, squatters and the mayor – was simply wild about Harry.

An interesting man and a pleasure to care for, one morning he asked me if I was familiar with the paintings of Peter Paul Rubens.

'No,' I said. 'Are you going to buy one?'

'I hadn't thought of it,' he said with a laugh, 'but you remind me of his models.'

221

I was quite flattered until I went to Dulwich Library and discovered that the women Rubens painted were on the 'robust' side and frequently starkers.

Revenge was mine on the day Harry's pretty secretary was sitting beside his bed. She was taking a letter and I asked her to leave so I could give her boss an injection.

'Are you going to stick a *huge* needle in his bottom?' she asked me, her eyes wide.

'Yes,' I said. 'And it's going to hurt like billy-o.'

'Then I'm staying,' she said firmly. 'I wouldn't miss this for the world.'

'Okay,' I said, grinning at her.

'Women!' Harry scoffed and turned on his side.

On the private wing, we also cared for Kurdish soldiers who had been injured fighting in the Middle East. Indigenous people of a vast mountainous region, the Kurds were essentially stateless; their numbers (in the millions) spread into Turkey, Iraq, Syria, Iran and Armenia. Our soldiers were mostly peasants and were well-mannered, appreciative and respectful towards English nurses.

A few had been without proper treatment for a while. On arrival, they were in a sorry state, with infected wounds and bedsores as deep as the ones I had seen at St Francis. We irrigated wounds and packed them with dressings to heal them from the inside out, and when the wounds showed no improvement using conventional treatments, we resorted to natural remedies. We had notable success, after infected matter and slough were removed, painting wounds with egg white, then drying them with a hairdryer.

One soldier I remember well. A handsome man in

his forties, with thick dark hair, a full moustache and eyes that seemed to dance when he smiled, he told us he was a general. His English was surprisingly good and his injury memorable: a bullet had shattered much of his right buttock, leaving a painful wound. It had not been gained on the battlefield; nothing so glorious. Our general informed us – with pride, I might add – that he had been discovered in bed with another general's wife and the other general had shot him in the backside. The opinion of the medical staff was that this was a cover story for having been shot while running away, but we nurses who cared for the general favoured the jealous-husband scenario.

General Mischief, as I called him, was nursed on his stomach until his wound had healed enough for him to walk around and sit pain-free on a commode chair with his injured bottom protruding through the seat. A warm, gregarious man, as soon as he was mobile he became a kind of cheer-up squad for other soldiers and was especially helpful to nurses and doctors when translation was needed. He even developed some useful instructions on how to use the sit-down toilet in the bathroom.

Our soldiers from rural areas had only ever seen and used a squat toilet (where you stand or squat over a hole in the floor) and were unfamiliar with Western-style sit-down toilets. Not long after General Mischief had translated to another soldier that I required a urine specimen, I found the soldier standing on the rim of the sit-down toilet. His pants were stretched to capacity between his ankles, his head and right hand pressed against the wall for balance. With his left hand, he was trying valiantly to capture some urine in the small pot, but most of it was splashing over his pants and feet.

Hearing the door, he swivelled his head so he could see me. 'Is okay, the general tell me how,' he said.

'That's good,' I said, and just managed to exit the bathroom before collapsing with laughter.

Hang on to your bonnets! The year 1974 marked a turning point for British nursing, and the speed of change was exhilarating.

I like to think that Bernice and I helped blaze the money trail with our rebellious resignations at the beginning of the year, mainly because our actions had elicited zero response at the time. But every little bit counts in a movement for change, and it wasn't long before other nurses made their feelings known.

Waving banners and chanting slogans, militant nurses marched en masse to 10 Downing Street and demanded better pay from Prime Minister Harold Wilson. In a shocking move, the normally staid Royal College of Nursing registered to become a trade union, and for the first time nurses in some parts of the country initiated strike action. Wards were closed and hospitals restricted to emergency admissions.

It was amazing. Even the medical profession voiced their support for our increased remuneration, and where nurses couldn't strike, coal miners offered to stop work on our behalf. Unbelievably, we won an average thirty per cent pay increase – an amount that was creeping towards a living wage. Imagine that!

Future career prospects were even more exciting. In response to the increasing use of technology, the expansion of transplant and cardiac surgery, and other advances in medicine and surgery, opportunities for nurses to specialize were springing up all over the place. In addition, the widespread establishment of identified units for intensive care, coronary care, and liver and kidney disease had also created further need for specialized nursing. With these changes came increased nurse responsibility for patient care and the possibility of improved and more diverse career structures.

Thanks to the 1972 Briggs Report, improvements in the education of student nurses and midwives were also starting to filter through, as well as the provision of further training in a range of disciplines for qualified nurses, not to mention the chance to qualify in the field of nurse education itself.

The year also saw the reorganization of the National Health Service and responsibility for the delivery of health and social services in the community transferring from the knitted-cardie brigade at the local council to newly established area health services. This completely changed the way health services were delivered in the community, and created demand for nurses specializing in many areas of family health, including family planning, immunization and child health.

Finally, the 1974 Health and Safety at Work Act provided more focus on the need for qualified personnel to oversee the health, safety and welfare of people in the workforce. Industrial nursing, or occupational health nursing, as it was also known, had been around in one form or another in industry for years, but the Act obliged many more organizations to employ nurses.

Nursing was on the launch pad, ready for take-off. And I like to think that, somewhere, Florence Nightingale and Edith Cavell were having one hell of a party.

CHAPTER 18

Shop!

Industrial Nursing, Selfridges, London: 1974–5

IT WAS A hot Saturday in August, almost noon, and I was lying on a towel in the back garden of our shared house in Beckwith Road. The lads upstairs were still asleep in their rooms, Alistair was in Nova Scotia on his medical locum, Jan was at work on Lonsdale, and Bernice was stomping up and down in the bath on her washing. Kathy had now married Dave, and we missed her dreadfully. It felt like a light had gone out.

Tired after a long stretch of night duty, I closed my eyes and imagined myself on the beach at Lindos, a heavenly Grecian sun warming my tanned face.

Suddenly, the French windows flew open and Bernice called, 'The lads and I are rowing in Dulwich Park. Do you want to come?'

Boating with Kip, Mark and Roman on a Saturday meant two things: there was no sport on television and someone would end up in the lake.

'Maybe another time,' I said, 'but thanks for asking.'

It would be fun, but I didn't trust myself in close proximity to Kip, especially while Alistair was in Nova Bloody Scotia. Since my mother's death, I'd been emotionally unstable and at risk of making stupid decisions. I was wisely avoiding Kip in case I abandoned propriety and threw myself at him.

I listened to my housemates' banter, thundering footsteps on the stairs and finally the front door slamming. Fully awake now, I turned to the 'Positions Vacant' page in *The Times*. Seeing as I was almost twenty-two and planned not to marry until I was thirty, it was time to undertake further training or find a permanent job with a regular income, holiday pay and sickness benefits. I couldn't go on living between London and Hindhead, and for my own sanity I needed to put some distance between myself and my father. Aunt Joan was taking a lot of weight off my shoulders, but it wasn't really her problem. I also thought it was time that Richard helped out. In fact, I had called him and told him so.

It was assumed by Richard that his medical career was more important than my nursing career, and it wasn't. Nobody was sending financial assistance my way, and I had to look out for myself. And let me tell you something else: because of concern for my father, I had decided not to go to Canada with Alistair, and had then learned, with a hefty dose of annoyance, that Richard and Esther were flying to Kenya for a safari! My dander up, I had told Richard that I fervently hoped he would be eaten by a lion. We hadn't spoken since.

One advertisement jumped off the page: a state registered nurse was required at Selfridges department store in Oxford Street.

I knew nothing about industrial nursing, but it might be worth trying for an interview. This type of job could have attractive benefits. And a small first-aid room where nothing much happened sounded like a good place to dip my toe into this type of nursing. I could already see the room – a table and two chairs (one for me and one for my patient), a first-aid box containing bandages and aspirin, a sink, an eye chart, a set of scales on the floor and a camp bed against the wall where an ailing shopper could lie down – and I would make tea and phone relatives and be ever so kind.

Minute by minute, the picture improved: regular hours, Sundays off, no night duty, no heavy lifting, staff discounts, and plenty of time to browse in the Pierre Cardin section at Miss Selfridge. The more I thought about it, the more the job had my name on it. I chose to ignore niggling concerns about IRA bombs.

With nothing to lose except the title of dutiful daughter, I gathered change, wandered down to the phone box at the end of the road and called the number listed. The woman who answered asked about my qualifications and experience. I made much of my King's training, obstetrics certificate and time in Casualty, and of what a jolly good first-aider I was.

An interview was arranged, and I hotfooted it to Dulwich Library for information on industrial nursing. Flicking through a book, I figured it all looked like common sense. The health and safety of employees at work was the primary focus, and it also involved protecting everyone from work-related hazards. (This was years before lawyers poked their noses in and health and safety became more concerned with protecting an employer from litigation than with actually looking after staff.)

I borrowed a St John Ambulance Brigade book in case, at the interview, there were questions about cuts and bruises, burns, sprains and other minor ailments.

Shop!

The big-ticket items – choking, heart attacks, strokes and broken legs – I knew well enough, but I couldn't imagine I would need to know about any of those.

Selfridges is a magnificent department store on Oxford Street, not far from Marble Arch. Along with its founder, Harry Selfridge, the store has been the co-star of the successful 2013 British television series *Mr Selfridge*.

For over a hundred years, people have flocked through the doors of the impressive neoclassical building that today employs several thousand staff and boasts the biggest beauty hall in the world. Famous for elaborate window displays, a high-end shopping experience and the innovative and, at times, controversial exhibitions, it's no surprise that Selfridges has been voted the world's best department store three times.

Back in 1974, the store was no less impressive when, with a mixture of nerves and excitement, I rode the escalators to the fifth floor for my interview in the first-aid room. On the way up, I stood behind a girl who was trailing a jet stream of the latest must-have perfume, Charlie. She had long blonde hair to her waist and was wearing a Laura Ashley dress. Around one tanned ankle was a silver bracelet laden with charms. I couldn't take my eyes off it. I *so* wanted to look like her. I *so* didn't look like her in my home-made green gabardine-cotton skirt, floral Dorothy Perkins blouse and sensible nursing shoes.

Each floor was a myriad of colours, lights, dazzling displays and beautiful people. There were staff everywhere assisting customers, as this was a time when staff were actually there to help you and not, as has become the case in many department stores,

229

merely lurking in the shadows to stop you helping yourself. The store was mesmerizing, and by the time I reached the fifth floor I wanted to work at Selfridges more than anything in the world.

My homely idea of a small first-aid room was a little off the mark. And it was apparent that the call for a nurse was not in response to recent health and safety legislation. I soon learned that the forward-thinking Mr Selfridge had insisted that a trained nurse be on hand from day one, back in March 1909. Over sixty years later, what was initially a first-aid room had expanded into a suite of treatment rooms that, according to the duty roster on the wall, had a doctor, three nurses, two dentists, a dental nurse and a podiatrist. Crikey!

Seated in the waiting area was a man in a white chef's coat. He was clutching a bloodied tea towel around his fingers. Next to him sat a girl with an angry stye under one eye; next to her was a man holding the side of his face. I was more than a trifle overwhelmed. No way would Selfridges be interested in inexperienced me. I was about to leave when a fine-boned, pretty girl of about my age walked around the corner and said, 'Hello, I'm Bambi, the senior nurse. Have you come for the interview?'

Caught before I could run, I swallowed and nodded. Her accent was Australian and she cocked her head a little to the side and smiled. 'Are you called Margaret?'

'Maggie,' I said, smiling back.

'Well, come with me, Maggie,' she said warmly, and I followed her to a treatment room that had a curtain for a door. She pulled the curtain for privacy and we sat opposite each other at the small table. Her movements, I noticed, were graceful and her manner gentle. She was well named.

Before asking questions, Bambi explained that in addition to providing emergency response to accidents in the store, the nurses treated minor staff ailments, made appointments with the doctor if necessary, carried out prescribed treatments, completed accident forms, monitored staff absence, assisted with rehabilitation following injury and return to work, provided pre-employment medicals, assessed a person's suitability to remain at work and ensured safety practices were followed in the workplace. There was a considerable workforce to be cared for, and the doctor, the dentists, the dental nurse and the podiatrist, she explained, were for staff, not customers. The nurses were for everybody.

I nodded enthusiastically. Bambi could have said I had to abseil down the outside of the building and clean the windows and I would still have wanted the job. But I knew the interview would be over once my lack of experience was raised.

'Can I see your certificates?' Bambi asked.

Sayonara, I thought.

I produced my King's certificate, my state registered nurse documents and my obstetrics certificate.

'These look in order,' she said, glancing over them. 'Have you any industrial nursing experience?'

'No,' I said, 'but I've worked in one of the world's busiest casualty departments at King's.'

'Anything else?'

I hesitated. 'Would the Girl Guides First Aid badge help?'

Bambi grinned. 'Not really.'

My spirits fell. She opened a folder and took out

stapled sheets of paper that appeared loaded with questions.

We completed name, age, address and qualifications. Great: we'd made page two. Bambi cleared her throat and looked through the remaining pages. Her nose screwed up in disapproval. 'Oh dear,' she said. 'This will take all day.'

I surmised the interview was over, but Bambi ploughed on – where was I born, my next of kin, relevant health history, languages spoken – and we were on page four when Bambi put down her pen and frowned. Perhaps she had realized, as I had, that there was no point in continuing. Slowly she closed the paperwork and leaned across the desk towards me.

'Look, Maggie,' she said, in a hushed, conspiratorial voice, 'do you want this job? Because you're the only person who has applied.'

For a second, I was taken aback. Then I saw a mischievous glint in her eyes and suddenly we were both laughing uncontrollably.

I was over the moon. I couldn't wait to write and tell Alistair that I had a proper job. To celebrate, I bought some Marks & Sparks knickers, David Bowie's *Diamond Dogs* LP and a Mars bar, which I devoured on the bus on the way home.

As I entered our front door, Kip was descending the stairs.

'Hello,' I said, and blushed. Fumbling with the shopping bags, I dropped my keys.

Kip picked them up and handed them to me. 'Why are you dressed like a librarian?'

'I've been for an interview at Selfridges.'

'And do they?'

'Do they what?'

'Sell fridges?' he said, and then he did it. He smiled.

Oh my god . . .

'No,' I blurted out, and hurried into my room. Shutting the door, I leaned hard against it and sighed. One can never be too careful with hormones.

I soon got into the swing of things at Selfridges and took great pleasure in realizing that my training, even though it hadn't specifically targeted industrial nursing, had prepared me well for it. Of course, I was learning new administrative requirements – referrals, accident forms, reports, treatment records, pre-employment medical forms and so on – and for the first two weeks, until I knew my way around the store, a security officer accompanied me and the trusty wheelchair to emergencies.

At any given time, there could be thousands of people in Selfridges and the adjacent Miss Selfridge. In addition to customers and sales staff, there were concession brand employees (mainly at cosmetics and perfume counters), kitchen staff, chefs and waiters, hairdressers, storemen, parking attendants, doormen, accountants, personnel staff, lift attendants, cleaners, delivery men, packers, security officers, telephonists and managerial staff, to name a few. Between them all, they managed to have at least one serious episode every few days: bad falls on escalators, nasty burns and lacerations in the kitchens, heavy boxes dropping on feet in the store room, choking in a restaurant, fingers smashed in car doors in the car park, broken arms and ankles from falling on the pavement outside, suspected heart attacks and strokes, and, my favourite, women going into labour in the menswear department.

Apart from Bambi and myself, the third nurse was Mary, a no-nonsense brunette from the north of England. The three of us worked well together. Bambi specialized in eyes, Mary was ears, and I was the star strapper and bandager, courtesy of the fracture clinic at King's. We supplied our own uniforms, and we worked five days a week, 8.50 a.m. to 5.50 p.m. (timed to cover staff entering and exiting the building outside shopping hours). The store was closed on Sundays, and Mary and I alternated working Saturdays so we had every second weekend off. The hours were brilliant.

Selfridges' medical officer, Dr Donald Page, held a surgery from Monday to Friday for staff. A debonair, grey-haired gentleman, he was also a Harley Street GP, and he was kind, thorough and delightfully eccentric. Older than time, or so he seemed to me, he wore a three-piece suit and a bowler hat to work every day and kept a never-ending cup of tea in the top drawer of his desk, from which he took sips between patients. Much to Mary's amusement, from the moment I arrived Dr Page called me Mary, or waved impatiently at me, saying, 'You, girl, come here,' as if I were keeping him waiting. Years later, I discovered he had been the staff doctor for MI5 during the Second World War.

Having a doctor, two dentists, three nurses and a podiatrist available for staff encouraged employees to attend to problems early. This prevented complications and allowed for regular treatment and follow-up without the loss of lengthy work hours. Minor ailments were our daily fare – sprained ankles, in-growing toenails, bunions, chilblains, diarrhoea, constipation, dermatitis, haemorrhoids, cystitis, acne, pregnancy, boils, colds, flu, headaches, rashes, coughs, varicose veins, blocked ears, styes, back strain, minor burns, splinters, perfume squirted in eyes, and unusual problems, like infected wounds between hairdressers' fingers and toes from tiny customer hairs that had penetrated their skin. We sent home the infectious, the genuinely unwell and anyone with a stomach upset who prepared food. One of the nurses (me) sent home a coughing and feverish parking attendant the day a Rolls-Royce was pinched from the car park. As it was my fault the car park had been left unattended, I was rather relieved when the poor chap was officially diagnosed with pneumonia.

Pre-employment medicals were also routine work. At the time, Selfridges was employing hard-working Ugandan Asians who had fled Africa in 1972 following President Idi Amin's dream that God had ordered him to expel all Asians. By 1974, many had made their way to England, but unfortunately about one in ten of the Selfridges applicants had pulmonary TB and required treatment before starting work. We kept the X-ray departments at nearby hospitals busy, I can tell you.

If there was an accident or medical emergency in the store, nurses were notified by telephone. Immediately, we took the first-aid bag and a wheelchair to the location, cleared the area and assessed the patient. For life-threatening incidents, treatment was commenced on site, an ambulance called and a security officer dispatched to meet the ambulance at the front door. For everything else, we applied immediate first aid, then escorted the person to the first-aid centre.

Occasionally, foreign 'customers' with a pre-existing medical condition pretended to be ill in the store, hopeful of receiving free treatment from the National Health Service. Also, drug addicts feigned collapse and renal colic, as they had in Casualty, searching for narcotics. But we were wise to all that malarkey.

Bomb threats to the store were an ever-present concern. The Provisional IRA had detonated bombs at Brooks's club in October and in a Woolwich pub in November, so we were prepared for evacuation and major trauma if the unthinkable happened. There was a specific sequence of overhead lighting throughout the store to alert staff that a bomb threat had been received. In response, staff would search their immediate area for an abandoned bag or package. If anything suspicious was found, the area would be evacuated until cleared by the Bomb Squad.

At Selfridges, we had our fair share of staff malingerers, many of whom were working their way through medical encyclopaedias in an effort to be sent home. They could have anything from leprosy to a headache in their elbow.

Their undisputed king was Roger the Dodger. Well over six foot, Dodger had a South London accent and the tallest Afro hairdo on earth. Clothes-wise, he favoured tight green tartan trousers, brown T-shirts, a multi-coloured jacket and brown, high-heeled platform boots – footwear that raised his height enough to register him with air-traffic control.

Dodger worked in the office at the delivery dock, although the word 'work' might be a stretch. Every day, his towering form loomed in the doorway of the first-aid centre with a new problem. His modus operandi never wavered. Unsteadily, he would make it to a chair and put the back of his hand to his forehead in melodramatic fashion.

'I got dust in me eye, you dig, man,' he told me one day. I gave him an eye bath and made a note of it.

'Can I go home now?' he asked afterwards.

'No!' I said.

Next it was, 'I gotta rash.' Diligently, I searched for a rash.

'It's rabies,' Dodger said.

'We don't have rabies in England,' I assured him, and dabbed calamine where he indicated a rash. As always, I made a note of it.

'Can I go home?' he asked.

Swallowing a laugh, I exclaimed, 'No!'

Then one day, Dodger arrived scratching his scalp with a ruler poked into his mass of hair. 'My head itches,' he complained.

'Stay there and don't sit down,' I ordered. If this was what I thought, I didn't want him sitting next to another patient. As Dodger was so tall, I went to find a stool to stand on. I met Bambi in the corridor and she grabbed a stool as well.

So there we were, two nurses standing on stools, peering into Dodger's hair when Dr Page opened his door. He was holding his teacup and looking for a refill.

'Head lice, is it?' Dr Page demanded.

Bambi and I nodded.

'Send him home!' Dr Page ordered.

'Bleedin' hell,' Dodger said. 'All this time, and all I had to do was scratch.'

During my time at Selfridges, the store was owned by the British financier and retail tycoon Sir Charles

Clore, or Charlie Boy, as we liked to call him. And Santa Clores at Christmas.

He was a wealthy man – and you've got serious money when you can name your oil tankers after your children – and his philanthropy was boundless. His financial support was behind many much-needed services in London, and there were buildings and even a beach named after this most generous of men, which is why, in the grand British tradition, it was fair game to safely take the mickey out of him for being cheap.

My favourite Charlie Boy story involved his purported exchange with a floorwalker in the menswear department. The world's most famous floorwalker was Captain Peacock from the seventies comedy series *Are You Being Served?* Employed by large stores, it was the floorwalker's job to oversee the staff in their department, assist customers and generally keep sales ticking over. It was a position to aspire to.

The story goes that Sir Charles was wandering through Selfridges when a floorwalker called Trevor, not knowing the owner's identity, approached him to ask if he needed assistance. Unfortunately, the sole on one of Trevor's shoes had come unstuck and was flapping up and down wildly as he walked.

'Your sole is falling off,' Sir Charles pointed out.

'I know, sir,' Trevor agreed. 'I haven't had time to repair it, and I can't afford another pair until payday.'

'Not to worry, son,' Sir Charles said and, delving into his pocket, he produced a roll of banknotes. Trevor's eyes were out on stalks.

Carefully Sir Charles removed the elastic band that was securely wrapped around the notes and held it out to the floorwalker. 'Here,' he said. 'Put this around your shoe. It'll hold the sole on until you can have it repaired.'

Christmas was coming and a tinselled Selfridges jingled to the sound of ringing tills and sleigh bells. Happy families flocked to see Santa and the dazzling Dickens-themed window displays that featured Oliver Twist and the like in a festive setting.

At times, it seemed all of London was in the store. On several occasions, there were so many shoppers that the doors had to be closed for everyone's safety. There were also bomb threats aimed at causing havoc during peak shopping hours, but thankfully no bombs were found. That is, until 19 December 1974, when the IRA detonated a massive time bomb in a parked car on Oxford Street outside Selfridges.

It was after closing time, management were holding their Christmas party on the top floor, and we nurses were on our way home. Not far away, musician Steve Lacy was performing at Wigmore Hall and Christmas shoppers were filling pubs and nearby restaurants.

The IRA gave three telephone warnings and the area was evacuated before the bomb exploded, thereby preventing many deaths and serious injuries. But no one knew about the management party at Selfridges. Why should they? It was assumed the store was empty, so the first that management knew of the bomb was when it exploded. Everybody was badly shaken by the blast, but the only injury I know of was a cut forehead.

I was already at home in Herne Hill when I heard the news about the bomb. I went numb. I'd been waiting at the bus stop on Oxford Street. And I had been on the bus when the bomb had exploded.

The next day, with a mixture of curiosity and apprehension, I went to work. Outside Selfridges, the explosion had ripped a huge hole in the road and caused enormous damage to the front of the store and the shops opposite. Oliver Twist and David Copperfield were goners. Windows and walls were blown out across a wide area of Oxford Street. But it was business as usual at Selfridges. Guided by police and doormen, I joined other staff as we gingerly picked our way past the devastation. Everyone stayed calm and carried on. It made me proud to be British.

Two days later, a hidden bomb was found by a vigilant staff member at Harrods in Knightsbridge. The store was evacuated, the bomb was defused and countless lives were saved.

My father and brother (who had not been eaten by a lion on safari, and with whom I was no longer cross) were both beside themselves with worry and wanted me to leave Selfridges.

'I'm staying and I'll be fine,' I reassured them – no way was I leaving before the January sales – but I was already reviewing other career options.

As a staff member I received a Selfridges discount booklet of coupons for forty per cent off clothes on top of the sales price, so it was time to pay for the Jaeger dress, skirt, cashmere sweater and leather coat that a salesgirl had put aside for me. (I still have the coat but it's a little tight. Actually, it doesn't fit me at all.)

There were other staff discounts on top of sales prices in the store, and I purchased a greenhouse for my father at a hefty discount that included delivery to Hindhead.

Shop!

In late January, I made an unannounced visit home. Herbie J had been happier lately and I wanted to make sure, for my own peace of mind, that his sobriety on my last visit had not been manufactured for my benefit.

It was dark when I walked up the driveway to the house. The garage door was open and I stepped through it to use the side door into the kitchen, taking note of my mother's old shopping basket on the freezer next to the car. In the basket were a bottle of wine, a newspaper folded to reveal the half-completed crossword, and my father's slippers.

Slippers? And the crossword that he always completed before switching off the bedside light?

I wandered into the kitchen, where Herbie J was writing a letter at the table.

'Hello, Maggie love,' he said, and smiled broadly. Relief flooded through me. The kitchen was tidy, my father was sober, his hair was combed, he was smartly dressed and he appeared happy. Fighting back tears, I kissed the top of his head. 'Thought I'd come down and help you put up the greenhouse,' I said.

'And make sure your father's not up to mischief?'

I smiled. 'That too. What's for dinner?'

'I'm picking up fish and chips on the way to Joan's. Do you want to come?'

'Love to,' I said. Aunt Joan lived in a lovely old house in West Liss.

Half an hour later, after a bath, I joined my father downstairs, and we locked up and climbed into his car. The basket was already on the back seat with the wine and an empty casserole dish. The slippers and the newspaper had been removed.

Ha! The old devil had been planning to stay the night with Joan!

Now, you might think this would upset me, but it didn't. My father had suddenly become someone else's responsibility and I felt a huge weight lifted off my shoulders. Although, when I thought about it, it was ridiculous that any dalliance was occurring between such old people. I mean, my father and Joan were in their fifties, for goodness' sake.

I looked sideways at my father and grinned.

'What?' he said, glancing at me as he pulled out of the driveway.

'Nothing,' I said.

Leaving Selfridges was a wrench, but for me there were too many bomb scares and one near miss. I adored the job and working with Bambi and Mary, but I knew that Bambi and her husband, Rod, would soon be returning to Australia. The job just wouldn't be the same without her.

On my last day at Selfridges, I emerged from the store to find the buses on strike, so I walked all the way home in the cold. It was a rather dismal finale to what had been the highlight of my career to date.

CHAPTER 19

A Country Practice

Haslemere and District Hospital, Surrey: 1975–6

'WHAT ARE ALISTAIR'S intentions?' my father asked me at the breakfast table. 'You've been together a long time.'

It was early May and I was in Hindhead for a couple of days to visit my father. The greenhouse looked dandy, as did my father. He and Aunt Joan had become a regular item on the Home Counties dating scene, and it suited me just fine. Instead of travelling frequently between London and Hindhead, I was now travelling frequently between London and Tunbridge Wells, which was where Kip, who had qualified as a doctor last year, was working as a houseman. I hadn't told my father that Alistair and I had parted company, or that I had resumed my relationship with Kip. Somehow I knew he wouldn't approve. I wasn't even sure that I approved myself.

'Intentions?' I asked casually.

Herbie J put down his mug of tea. 'You're not making it easy for Alistair, are you, Maggie love?'

Amused by his rather ham-fisted way of asking whether Alistair and I were sleeping together, I replied,

'Mum would have told you that I never made anything easy for anyone.'

He smiled at the thought. 'You know perfectly well what I mean.'

'I do,' I said, 'and I'm going to work.' I stood up and threw him a look that said, 'Quit while you're ahead.' Escaping the kitchen, I went to my room and packed, ready to return to London.

Since leaving Selfridges, I'd been working as an agency staff nurse, mostly, would you believe, on Dickens at St Giles. Sister Morag had long gone and there was a healthier atmosphere on the ward. For me, though, every corner of Dickens brought flashbacks of anguish, which was why, as agency Staff Nurse Johnson, I made an effort to treat student nurses with kindness and respect, and to ensure there was a fair division of labour and learning. Not a day went by on Dickens when I didn't shudder to recall how close I had been to throwing in the towel during those early months of my own training.

It's true that I was missing the glamour and excitement of Selfridges, but, as I told Bambi, working as an agency staff nurse and banking higher wages fitted my grand plan. I had written to the King Edward VII Memorial Hospital in Bermuda enquiring about a position and was awaiting a reply. Everything about the island – the climate, the pink-sand beaches and the coral reefs – appealed to me. Bermuda, I'd decided, would be my stepping stone to Australia.

Apart from accumulating funds, there was something else I wanted to do before going abroad. Ever since my interview to train at King's, I had dreamed of working in a village hospital in rural England – or, to be precise, the old gabled building at the end of a sweeping drive lined with flowering roses that I had wrongly imagined King's would be. I wanted to be the nurse I'd pictured pushing an injured soldier in a wheelchair across a lawn, and I knew I would find such a hospital if I kept looking.

By summer, Kip and I had parted company *again* (honestly, we were more exciting than Burton and Taylor) and my grand plan was in tatters. There was no reply from Bermuda and I'd spent all my savings on a holiday in Greece with Jan and Bernice. And as for finding my dream village hospital, there was no hope of that if I stayed in London.

Despondent, I had a complete meltdown and left London, running home to Hindhead, where I sat like a dispirited lump at the kitchen table and told my startled father what a loser I was – jobless, dateless, broke and living at home at twenty-two.

'You've only been here two hours,' he pointed out.

'Well, it feels like for ever,' I grumbled uncharitably.

Herbie J let me stew for three days and then, on the ruse of cheering me up with a country drive, my shrewd remaining parent pulled over outside a farm gate on which a notice was pinned: FRUIT PICKERS WANTED. APPLY WITHIN.

'Will you look at that!' he said, as if it was the first time he'd seen the sign.

Frowning, I got out of the car and applied within.

'You'll do,' the farmer said.

The dew was still on the ground when I started work in the fields the following morning. For much of July, I picked raspberries and blackcurrants every day, slowly healing with the country air in my lungs and the warm summer sun on my back. I worked hard and relished being alone with my thoughts and the sounds of nature. And I would probably still be there if the nursing agency hadn't called to ask if I could work a few shifts on a female ward at a small hospital in Haslemere. They were desperate, which meant hard physical work was involved.

'What does the hospital look like?' I asked the woman at the agency.

'It looks like a hospital,' she said impatiently.

Realizing she must think I'd been at the Scotch, I accepted the work and explained the situation to the farmer.

'Good Lord,' he said, raising his eyebrows. 'You don't look anything like a nurse!'

And I didn't. Tanned and wild-looking in a torn T-shirt and frayed denim shorts, I had strands of sun-bleached hair poking out from under a tatty straw hat, berry juice stains on my hands and knees, scratches on my arms and legs, and solid mud caking my sensible nursing shoes.

Laughing at his surprise, I said, 'You don't know how happy I am to hear you say that.'

It was obviously my week for the firmament to bestow unexpected delights. Alistair wrote to me and we rekindled our relationship. And my father bought me a second-hand Mini Clubman, seeing that I was prepared to work hard. Harvest Gold was the colour. Goldie was the name.

'I bought your brother a sports car before he went to university,' he told me, as if I hadn't noticed that I'd been given a suitcase before I went nursing. 'You didn't need a car in London,' he went on, 'but you need one now.' I didn't dare ask why he hadn't bought me a new Austin-Healey Sprite.

But I did need a car, and I was grateful. My father was driving me to the farm every day, and I disliked being dependent on him. For an hour, I sat in Goldie in the garage and practised getting in and out, locking the door and walking casually away, a sophisticated, happening girl-about-town. The garage backdrop wasn't really working for me, so I drove into Guildford and did the same thing in the high street. It worked much better there.

Driving along Church Lane and pulling up at Haslemere and District Hospital is a lasting memory. On climbing out of the car, I stood near a bed of roses and stared at the old gable-roofed brick-and-shingle building. Over the years, unattractive extensions had been added here and there, but that didn't take away the magic. My eyes saw only what they wanted to see: the village hospital of my dreams. And, if I thought hard, I could picture myself pushing an injured soldier in a wheelchair across a lawn.

A relieved Sister Lambert greeted me warmly when I walked on to Elizabeth ward for my first morning shift. A capable-looking woman in her late forties, with tightly permed white hair, Sister Lambert was exhausted. I quickly learned that she hadn't had a day off since ... She couldn't remember when. Apparently, no one had replaced the staff nurse who had left.

Considerably smaller than the Nightingale wards I was used to in London, Elizabeth ward was bright and airy, and the sky and treetops visible through the open windows bestowed a bucolic feeling of rural calm. There were vases of home-grown dahlias on bed-tables, and the strong scent of 4711 in the air – 'the cologne from Cologne', as my grandmother had called it.

The majority of female patients on the ward were elderly, with a range of medical problems – angina, hypertension, congestive cardiac failure, emphysema, peptic ulcer, pleurisy, stroke – all of which required specific treatments in addition to basic nursing care. Some patients, following hip surgery in Guildford, had been transferred to Elizabeth ward to recuperate. Others were awaiting a bed at a nursing home.

The morning went by in a flash. Sister Lambert and I, helped by three nursing assistants, worked hard. As I'd expected, there was a lot of heavy lifting, but after a month of picking fruit, my back was as strong as an ox's.

Physiotherapists came and went, and local GPs wandered in willy-nilly to see their patients. Unlike the doctors I was used to in London, the country GPs did not expect nurses to stop what they were doing and run to their side. It struck me that they were far more respectful of the nursing profession, seeking our opinions and responding to requests with constructive discussion before changing medications and ordering tests.

At noon, dead on her feet, Sister Lambert asked if I could run the ward if she went home to rest for a few hours. By the end of my King's training, I had been capable of running a general ward, so I confidently told her to go home. At Haslemere, many nurses worked split shifts – starting early in the morning, leaving at noon, then returning in the early evening – to cover the busiest times on the wards. Afternoons were reserved for patients' rest time and visiting hours, and were often staffed by a qualified nurse and a nursing assistant, namely myself and a girl called Hope on that first day.

Not half an hour after Sister Lambert had left, a GP admitted Mrs Lorna Adams, a forty-year-old woman with a crippling headache. The GP suspected migraine and ordered pethidine. When his patient was settled, he left instructions to call him if her condition changed. Mr Adams, who arrived soon after his wife, sat beside her bed looking worried.

A short time later, Mrs Adams started vomiting, her neck stiffened, her pulse slowed and she began drifting in and out of consciousness. I called the GP, but he was on his rounds, so I left a message for him to come urgently to the hospital. Then I called the switchboard to page any doctor in the hospital to come to Elizabeth ward.

The only doctor was busy with another seriously ill patient and couldn't come. Oh, what to do? I suspected Mrs Adams was having a cerebral aneurysm and, if I was right, there was no time to waste. Could Haslemere deal with this? I had no idea of the hospital's capabilities. Was it mad to call an ambulance to a hospital?

At King's, I was taught always to put the patient first, which made my decision easy. Mrs Adams needed to be transferred to a bigger hospital where I *knew* there were resources to care for her. I called an ambulance, then phoned the Royal Surrey County Hospital in Guildford, which wasn't far away, and advised them of Mrs Adams's symptoms and that the patient would soon be on her way.

The GP and the ambulance officers arrived on the ward together, and I readied myself for backlash from the GP. Instead he said, 'Good call, Nurse,' and he went in the ambulance with Mrs Adams and her husband to Guildford, bells ringing as it sped away.

By the time Sister Lambert returned in the late afternoon, radio-opaque dye had been injected into Mrs Adams's carotid artery at Guildford Hospital and an aneurysm diagnosed. She was being transferred to London for surgery, which we later learned was successful.

For my part, I had inadvertently secured future employment as an agency nurse at Haslemere and District Hospital for as long as I wanted. And I wanted it very much.

I quickly discovered the source of the 4711 cologne from Cologne. At the entrance to Elizabeth was a room with curtained windows that provided a view of the ward. Usually reserved for infectious patients or those nearing the end of life, on Elizabeth the room was the domain of Mrs Keats, a pleasant and decidedly large bedridden elderly lady who was the mother of a local councillor.

I discovered that in a country hospital the mother of anyone on the council is akin to royalty, and royally Mrs Keats behaved and royally she was treated. I have absolutely no idea what was wrong with her except that she was unable to walk. But she could talk. Boy, could she talk. And not once in the many months I looked after her did I hear her say a bad word about anyone except the prime minister, Harold Wilson. And he received a great many tongue-lashings.

We nursed Mrs Keats on a heated waterbed, and I

have warm memories of her wearing a voluminous shower cap and bobbing about like a cork on a pond between Hope and me as we changed the sheets without lifting her out. At times, the poor woman must have felt seasick from it all, but she never complained. I don't recall ever seeing her out of bed, but she received such excellent care that there wasn't a bedsore in sight.

At mealtimes, Mrs Keats preferred her napkin folded just so, and her water glass on the tray, not on the bedside locker. For afternoon tea, she favoured strawberry jam sandwiches that had been chilled in the fridge for an hour. Not one of the nurses begrudged Mrs Keats her special treatment, but the patients, many of whom knew each other and knew Mrs Keats, were infected with petty jealousies.

'What's so special about her?' they complained.

'Special?' I said, feigning ignorance.

'Is she paying or something?' they wondered.

'Of course not!' I told them.

Many of the ambulant patients sat and talked to bed-bound women. Gravitating towards others with a similar illness, they became informal support groups before such things had a name. They helped with flowers and at mealtimes, but no one went near Mrs Keats. Ironically, her royal place in the town's hierarchy had isolated her, and with our special attentions we nurses had condemned her to loneliness. It was, I think, a high price to pay for the trappings of privilege.

In August 1975, almost two years after my mother's death, my father married my aunt Joan at a small register-office ceremony. There were a few guests, including me, Joan's daughter Suzie and her husband,

John, and their two daughters. My brother couldn't attend, but on the upside, Suzie, who had been our second cousin, was now also our step-sister. I'd always wanted a sister.

Alistair and I were wearing out tyres travelling up and down the A3 to see each other. Sometimes we met in Brighton or spent the weekend at a friend's house in Kent, and at others he stayed with me in Hindhead. Life in rural England was good and I felt no urgent need to move back to London, even though the tedium of having napkins with every meal was starting to pall. But I'm being ungrateful. Living with my father and Aunt Joan was comfortable, and, even allowing for rent and board, I was saving well. And having spent most of my life separated from my father when he was at sea, I was cherishing the time with him. During those months at Hindhead we did, I suppose, get to know each other.

I enjoyed working on Elizabeth ward immensely. The staff were friendly and I revelled in the responsibility I was given. I never pushed an injured soldier in a wheelchair across a lawn, but I gained an insight into small-town politics in provincial Britain. And I began to respect the viewpoints of people from all walks of life, however salient or nuts they were.

From the old ladies, I learned that while everyone wanted to live a long life, no one wanted to be old; that old bones ached when it rained; that arthritis was worse if you swallowed too many tomatoes; and that rubbing a sore old muscle with a piece of ice wrapped in gauze numbed the area prior to an injection. I have fond memories of Mrs Percival (pneumonia) teaching me to crochet, Mrs Watson (hip replacement) teaching me to thread a needle by putting the needle on to the cotton instead of trying to push the cotton through the needle, and of Beryl the kitchen maid showing me how to make a proper sandwich with the butter spread right to the crusts. 'You could grow another arm with the goodness of my sandwiches, Maggie,' she told me.

Country folk, I discovered, have a strong sense of ownership of their local hospital. Their forebears fought to build the facility, generations were born or had given birth there, many raised funds to provide much-needed equipment, a fair few pushed the library trolley and volunteered their time, and many had friends and relatives who worked there. It was woe betide the cold-hearted bureaucrat who attempted to close the hospital or reduce services, for out they'd come with their furled brollies shaking in the air, marching as to war.

The start of 1976 brought opportunities for change. The BNA asked me if I was interested in working at a university hospital in Lausanne, a town on Lake Geneva in the French-speaking part of Switzerland. My schoolgirl French was rusty, and the agency offered an intensive French course in London to bring me up to scratch. It was tempting. I had money in the bank, the village hospital part of my grand plan was completed, and I was ready to travel abroad. Bermuda still hadn't replied to my application, so I accepted the Swiss offer.

At the beginning of February, my father sold our family home, Talisman, in Hindhead and moved into Joan's beautiful old house in West Liss. A few hundred years old, the house had originally been tithe cottages. It was as pretty as a picture on a chocolate box.

As soon as the move was over and my father settled, I said goodbye to country life. Leaving Elizabeth ward was a weepy affair, and I was truly touched when my colleagues presented me with an engraved fob watch. We hugged. We'd miss each other. We'd write. We never did.

I packed Goldie and moved back to an obscenely cold and grey winter in London, where I stayed with Alistair at his late aunt's house in Edgware Road, near Selfridges. Bambi and her husband, Rod, had already returned to Australia, but Jan and Bernice were still in London, both working at King's. Miranda was married and working as a health visitor, Polly had married and moved abroad, and Meredith and I were still exchanging letters between Canada and England. Jan and I visited Kathy and Dave in Birmingham and it was wonderful to see Kathy so happy and contented. Somehow, as with Laurel and Tilly, I had lost contact with Adele and Fraser.

In London, I threw myself into the language course and everything Swiss. I took the tube to Swiss Cottage, a London suburb named after a pub that looked like a Swiss cottage. I found the pub and went inside for a drink.

'A lot of nurses from the Royal Free come in here,' the barman said. He placed my gin and tonic on the bar.

'Oh, I'm not a nurse,' I said firmly.

'You sure look like one,' he said.

'I'm not,' I insisted.

He looked doubtful. Then he looked thoughtful. Finally, he said, 'Nah, give over, you're pulling my leg,' and went to serve someone else.

At Alistair's, I listened to records by Jacques Brel

(Belgian) and Michel Sardou (French). I munched my way through a barrel of Lindt chocolates (Swiss) while watching French films. And I started speaking English with a heavy French accent.

Two weeks after starting the language course, and a week after I had spent a fortune on a fabulous pair of calf-hide snow boots, a letter arrived from the King Edward VII Memorial Hospital in Bermuda offering me a job as a registered nurse. Attached to it was a colourful brochure with tropical-themed pictures of palm trees, blue sky and sandy beaches.

The Gods too, it seemed, were fond of a joke.

CHAPTER 20

There's No Business Like Snow Business

Centre Hospitalier Universitaire Vaudois and Hôpital Sandoz, Lausanne, Switzerland: 1976–7

SOME PEOPLE SAY that when you come to a fork in the road, you should take it, and that was how I felt about Switzerland and Bermuda. I wanted to experience both. Alistair didn't want me to do either and neither did my father. But Aunt Joan said I wasn't to live by others' wishes and to 'just do it'. So I did. And I went to Switzerland because I could take my car and it was easier to come home if I didn't like it.

As soon as the French course finished, I packed Goldie with essentials – cushions, teapots, books, sherry glasses, Toulouse-Lautrec posters, a porcelain umbrella stand (don't ask), Eddie Bear and my nurse uniforms – and said goodbye to family and friends.

'*Bon voyage!*' they yelled, as I set off for Dover, with Alistair for company on the trip.

'*Au revoir!*' I shouted back enthusiastically, oblivious to my father's sadness at my leaving England, just as I imagined he had been blind to my sorrow when he had left home to sail the seven seas throughout my childhood.

Taking turns, we drove through a sleepy France towards Switzerland, and as long as I live I will never forget my first sight of Lausanne, the university city on the northern shores of Lake Geneva that was to be my new home. Built on a hillside and wearing a dusting of late winter snow, the old red-roofed buildings were dominated by the spire and carved portals of a large Gothic cathedral. Towards the south, early morning sunlight danced on the lake against a distant landscape of snow-covered peaks that looked like a giant Toblerone with icing sugar on top. It took my breath away.

Later, after a lakeside picnic of baguette, Emmental and wine, I deposited Alistair at the station to catch the train home. It was a teary goodbye. Alistair would be over again in a few weeks and I would write every day. But somehow that didn't work out, and as my brother told my father (who then told me), another good man had had a lucky escape. For what it's worth, Alistair settled in America as an eminent physician and a professor at a famous university medical school. I know, don't say it. He could have done so much better if he'd stayed with me.

Anxious that I was suddenly alone in Europe, I kept busy and drove to the Centre Hospitalier Universitaire Vaudois (CHUV – pronounced Shoov), the teaching hospital where I would be working. Pulling up outside, I stared at the impressive multi-storey building and felt a sudden rush of excitement. Or was it nerves? CHUV was bigger than I had anticipated . . .

Dismissing unhelpful thoughts, I found an international telephone exchange and called my father.

'Much snow on the roads?' he asked.

'Hardly any,' I told him.

'It's raining here,' he said, 'and more expected tomorrow.'

Twenty francs a minute and the English talk about precipitation.

Daughter duties completed, I drove to Pont-de-Chailly and moved into the studio apartment organized by the hospital. In no time I had the place looking like a bazaar, with draped Oriental fabrics, posters on walls and plants in brass pots. I had just filled the fridge with groceries when there was a knock at my door.

'Hello, I'm Maya, your neighbour,' said the pretty dark-haired girl standing in the hallway. 'I'm a physio at Hôpital Sandoz. Are you the nurse who's going to work at CHUV?' I nodded and smiled. Maya had an American accent, freckles across her tanned face, and she was holding a marvellous-looking chocolate cake.

'Welcome to Switzerland!' she said brightly.

Wearing a badge bearing the unfamiliar title MADEMOISELLE JOHNSON, I felt like an impostor when I started work as an *infirmière* (nurse) on the neurosurgical intensive-care unit at CHUV. Thrown in at the deep end, I specialled an unconscious woman who'd had part of her skull removed to relieve pressure on her brain. You couldn't see her for tubes and bandages, but I knew that somewhere in there was a much-loved wife and mother called Gislaine.

On the unit a qualified nurse was allocated to each high-dependency patient and the atmosphere was intense. Doctors and nurses talked constantly against a backdrop of bright lights, beeping machines and phones ringing with pathology results. In contrast, the patients rarely made a sound. Sedated or unconscious, some had infections or injuries to the brain, spinal cord or nerves, while others had neurological diseases. Most were being treated and monitored either prior to surgery or post-operatively.

Assuming it was beneficial to practise French on a native speaker who couldn't laugh at my accent, I continually informed Gislaine of what I was doing as I checked her vital signs, fluid levels and neurological responses. Every change in her condition had to be reported. Nothing was left to chance. Life in the unit was fragile, and hope could give way to hopelessness in a heartbeat. We were all aware the Grim Reaper stalked the corridor outside, and not just for patients. During my first week, one of the doctors threw himself off a bridge.

The unit was plunged into a bleak sadness, and the grief of those who had known him was questioning and raw. Had he told anyone what was wrong? Why hadn't he?

Tragedy casts a net of doubt over everything, and I found myself wondering if coming to Switzerland had been a mistake. The big wide world was proving too big, too alien, but thankfully good sense prevailed. I had hardly known the man and had no right to hijack grief for self-indulgent purposes, so I pulled myself together and occupied my mind and time caring for Gislaine.

Most of the nursing staff were British and I soon became pals with Stella, a petite Yorkshire lass and senior nurse. The medical team included doctors from different countries and the shared experience and knowledge made ward rounds genuinely interesting. Communication was mainly in French, although we British girls lapsed easily into English when working together. Switzerland boasts four official languages, German, French, Italian and Romansh, and many staff were multi-lingual.

School French and the language course were serving me well, but I was having problems with the subtle nuances of Swiss-French and the tongue-twister name of the unit that had to be announced each time the phone rang. Taking a deep breath, I would pick up the phone and say, '*Allo, Centre Hospitalier Universitaire Vaudois, neurochirurgie soins intensifs, qui est à l'appareil?*' And honestly, by the time I'd said all that the edelweiss were out.

The caller would then bark something unintelligible involving numbers – counting is slightly different in Swiss-French – and I would pass the receiver to the nearest person and say, 'It's for you.'

Attached to the unit was a tall, thirty-something Greek psychiatrist, and it had not escaped my notice that he was attractive in a Zhivago kind of way. His name was Petros and one morning he suggested I simply say, '*Allo,*' when answering the phone. Then he invited me to lunch by the lake at Ouchy and, smiling demurely, I accepted.

Arriving at the restaurant, I discovered that Petros had also invited Stella and other doctors and nurses, and I soon realized the lunch was a much-needed morale boost for the team. Annoyed for conceitedly thinking it was a date, I nevertheless felt happy to be included and discovered that, away from work, formalities were dropped and my colleagues were relaxed and fun.

A week after the Ouchy lunch, Petros invited me to lunch at Chillon near Montreux. Again I accepted, only this time it was different.

'Where are the others?' I asked him when I arrived at the restaurant. Petros was sitting at a table for two on a terrace that extended over Lake Geneva. Sunlight was shimmering on the water behind him.

Grinning, he shrugged and said mischievously, 'I didn't ask them.'

My legs a little wobbly, I sat down.

Those long leisurely lunches at Chillon and at the old brasseries in Lausanne were to become a regular event that summer for me and Petros. I was to discover the wonders of Byzantine art, the pleasure of music by Theodorakis and books by Kazantzakis, and the joy of cartoons by Sempé.

Apart from chocolate, watches, banks, gnomes, the Red Cross, cow bells and objections to war, the Swiss have had other good ideas. For a start, making hospital beds was a breeze. Instead of a sheet and blankets, a warm, lightweight duvet covered the patient. It was much simpler than all that British hospital-corner business. Another winner was the *poste pneumatique*, a network of narrow pipes extending throughout the hospital that propelled capsules to their destination by compressed air. The sender placed pathology specimens, medicines, pharmacy requests and so on in the capsule, selected the destination's number and sent it on its way. Brilliant!

Work on the unit involved high levels of stress, and even though I enjoyed working with Stella, Petros and the team, I was experiencing the same problem I'd had in operating theatres during my training: I preferred patients who were awake and could communicate. Also, my French wasn't going to improve unless I was using it all the time, and there was no hope of that if I was working with nurses who frequently spoke English and patients who couldn't speak at all.

My request to transfer was approved and I accepted a nursing position across the road at Hôpital Sandoz, where my neighbour, Maya, worked as a physio.

'Good luck at Sandoz with Madame Durig,' a doctor warned me. 'You'll need it.'

I smirked. No one could ever be as bad as Sister Morag at St Giles.

Madame Durig at Hôpital Sandoz was as mad as a cut snake. An uncoordinated, sweaty, angry-faced skeleton of a woman – and that's just her good points – she was a Swiss-German nurse who revelled in her position of importance as a native Swiss.

As the newest Sandoz recruit, I was mildly fearful to learn that Durig had developed a taste for making life unpleasant for my British compatriots, Victoria and Blythe on the first floor, and Pippa on the second. Her arsenal included unpleasant comments about their French accents, threats over perceived wrongdoings (no one knew what they were), accusations of formal complaints (again, no one knew what they were) and belittling over imaginary misdeeds in front of patients, visitors and doctors.

This behaviour was absurd as all three girls were terrific, hard-working nurses. Victoria was a striking, sophisticated, dark-haired girl who took no notice of

Durig's hurtful comments, which infuriated the old bat. Blythe was a sweet-faced red-head from the north of England who was not averse to giving Durig a good verbal fight. And Pippa was our Alice in Wonderland, complete with long blonde hair, an Alice band and the sweetest disposition on earth. Pippa was the target of Durig's most vicious verbal attacks – until I arrived and she smelt fresh blood. But if Durig's plan was to divide and conquer the British, it went awry. Instead, our shared misfortune forged strong friendships between Victoria, Blythe, Pippa and myself.

Sandoz was a small hospital that specialized in physical medicine and rehabilitation – anything to do with bones, brain and spinal injuries, muscle damage and stroke recovery. Gislaine, whom I had nursed on the neurosurgical unit, was also on our floor. She had suffered a stroke and been transferred to Sandoz for rehabilitation, and was recovering well. It was good to talk with the real Gislaine, and I asked if my voice sounded familiar, but it didn't.

Each ward at Sandoz covered an entire floor and was known by its level in the building rather than a name. My floor, the *troisième étage*, was the third and top floor. A very wide corridor separated the nurses' office, kitchen, bathrooms and utility rooms from the patients' single and multi-bed rooms on the other side.

One day I was standing in the corridor, talking on the wall phone to a patient's relative, when Madame Durig appeared out of nowhere, walked up to me and said viciously, 'Rost beef!' Then she swiped me round the head before walking on.

'Hey!' I yelled, and she wheeled around looking shocked, either genuinely alarmed at what she had done or horrified that her action had been witnessed by a Czechoslovakian doctor who had just rounded the top of the stairs.

The obvious response was to report the incident, but to whom? And would they believe two foreigners? So I did nothing, and the longer I did nothing the more Durig stayed away from me. Mutual fear had been established and Durig, frightened to the depths of her racist soul that I still might report the matter, rarely spoke to me after that. It still stands as the only time in my life I have been hit – a surprise when you think about it.

On the *troisième étage*, we were lucky to have the glamorous Madame Kaspar, a Czech nursing sister, in charge. A tall, thirtyish, competent woman with swinging shoulder-length hair and a flirtatious disposition, she had escaped her homeland in 1968 with her husband and settled in Switzerland. In addition to Kaspar and myself there was an efficient Swiss-French nurse, Mademoiselle Bossard, who moved at warp speed and ate three apples a day. If there were other nurses, I don't remember them, but bringing up the rear as nursing aides was a happy bunch of nicely rounded Portuguese ladies, who were kind, thoughtful and moved very slowly. Always smiling, they reached out and lightly touched whoever they were talking to. I adored them.

We all pitched in with the physical workload of preparing patients for their morning physio, and Kaspar and I shared responsibility for medications, surgical dressings and doctors' rounds. Instead of a bath or shower, our patients preferred to perform their ablutions in bed in the form of a self-administered bed-bath. With great care, they gently washed and dried themselves, using two bowls of hot water on the bed-table, soap, a washcloth and a couple of towels. Nurses were then called in to wash backs and feet, after which the patients lovingly anointed themselves with a skin tonic called Bien-Être. This long-winded and leisurely coddling was a perfect example of the enviable French attention to self, and it made patients feel good, both physically and mentally. Sadly, the British are inoculated at birth against such self-indulgent pampering.

Coming from seventies Britain, I was also accustomed to egotistical doctors denouncing alternative health treatments and accusing its practitioners of quackery. It was refreshing to find the conservative Swiss embracing the health benefits of nature's bounty, with natural remedies administered as an adjunct to modern medicine in a hospital setting.

At Sandoz we made poultices of wild cherry bark to draw boils, and brewed tisane infusions of dandelion, lavender, raspberry, mint, lemongrass, ginger and chamomile to assist a range of problems. Tisanes were delivered daily on a trolley, and some patients drank a cup for health reasons while others simply enjoyed the occasion. Personally, I thought it all tasted like boiled straw with a dash of lemon disinfectant, but I never let on.

I should also tell you about the drinks trolley that rattled around the *troisième étage* at dinner time. Most patients had their own labelled bottle of Swiss wine from which they drank a glass with their meal, and this may explain how the Swiss manage to consume almost their entire wine production by themselves.

*

Because everything in Switzerland runs like clock-work, and there is nothing to grumble about, the Swiss have taken a lead from the French and become end-lessly paranoid about draughts. In hushed tones they speak of a *courant d'air* and move furniture about for fear of sitting between a door and a window. I was to discover that it wasn't only minor air currents that worried them . . .

'Do you know why this patient's shoulder surgery has been cancelled?' I asked a doctor.

'It's the Foehn,' he replied casually. 'The surgeon won't operate until it's blown through.'

'Of course,' I said. 'I should have realized.'

Later, I telephoned Petros. 'What's the Foehn?'

He chuckled. 'It's a warm wind in the Alps, and it makes everything go wrong. Even Swiss trains arrive two minutes late when the Foehn blows.'

'You're not serious?' I said.

'Quite serious,' he assured me. 'It turns honest people into bank robbers, and patients having minor ops have been known to die unexpectedly.'

'So it's a superstition,' I said, incredulous.

'More a respected legend,' Petros advised.

So I respected it, and whether it was bad juju or not, the patients didn't sleep well when the Foehn blew, and neither did I. But I probably would have slept better had I known of the Swiss contingency plans against other nasties that could be carried on an ill wind.

One afternoon at work I threw out medications past their expiry date and completed an order form to replace everything. I left the form for Madame Kaspar to add to if she thought of anything else we needed.

The following day I saw that she had doubled the quantities. Intrigued, I asked why.

'If things have expired up here,' she said, 'they will have expired downstairs.'

Assuming she was referring to the lower floors, I said, 'But they place their own orders.'

'No, I mean below Sandoz,' she elaborated. 'Everything has to be replaced down there too.'

Another ward below Sandoz? What on earth was she talking about?

Registering my confusion, Kaspar explained that below ground Switzerland has enough nuclear fallout facilities to accommodate the entire population. Complete with ventilation and anti-gas filters, every shop, cinema, hospital, school, home and mountain chalet has a reinforced steel door leading to a fallout facility.

'Even the patisserie?' I asked.

She nodded. 'Even the patisserie.'

In the event of a nuclear attack the rest of Europe would perish, but all the macaroons in Switzerland would be perfectly safe.

Throughout winter a steady stream of patients was admitted to Sandoz for rehabilitation following accidents in snow and ice. Swiss roads were regularly cleared and most vehicle mishaps were due to speed in poor conditions. Apart from car crashes, elderly folk slipped on ice and fractured femurs, and skiers and speed skaters challenged nature head-on and broke just about everything else.

Each morning, before Maya and her team of physiotherapists arrived on the ward, patients awaiting therapy sat on stools in the bathroom and dangled their legs in a hydro tub of warm water to loosen their muscles. But there was one patient we couldn't get into the bathroom: Madame Rosa Rostova.

A tiny mouse-like woman with bird's-nest hair, Rosa was Russian, seventy-six and had survived internment in a German concentration camp during the Second World War. She lived alone in the Swiss mountains, had fallen on ice and been found on a trail by cross-country skiers. Suffering from hypothermia and a fractured ankle, Rosa was admitted to Sandoz for nursing care and rehabilitation. Except she wasn't having any part of our nursing care and rehabilitation.

Rosa screamed and hollered when nurses entered her room, covered her head with her arms when meals were served, and shouted Russian obscenities at Maya and other physios. And, oh, joy of joys, she screeched blue murder at Madame Durig. I had the pleasure of acting surprised. 'I can't imagine what's got into her,' I said to a startled Durig. 'Rosa's never done that to anyone else.'

Enter Petros, the psychiatrist. As soon as he walked into her room, Madame Rostova threw a pillow at him. This was closely followed by a tissue box and a shoe. I didn't see any more because I left and closed the door. A while later, Petros emerged. Rosa's behaviour, he thought, might be related to trauma associated with filth in the concentration camp. He suggested that no Swiss-German or German enter her room, and that I place disposable gloves, a bowl of hot water, a flannel, soap and a towel on her bed-table and see what she did with them.

Looking worried, the Portuguese nursing aides watched as I gingerly entered the room and placed the bowl of water and other items on Rosa's bed-table.

They all smiled as I emerged empty-handed and dry. We listened for a crash. Nothing. We huddled around the door and shortly heard the trickle of water.

'She's wringing out the flannel,' I guessed and opened the door for a peek. Wearing disposable gloves, Madame Rostova was washing herself, her tongue protruding with concentration. She glanced towards the door and I quickly smiled.

'*Anglaise*?' she asked, and I nodded.

'Okay,' she said, and carried on washing herself.

Withdrawing, I carefully closed the door.

From then on Madame Rostova wore gloves to wash herself, which she did about twenty times a day, always putting on clean gloves to eat her meals. Doctors, nurses and physios wore gloves in her presence, and as the cleaner was Swiss-German, I cleaned Rosa's room myself.

It transpired that she could speak only a little French, so we communicated with her by using picture boards and mime, a bit like charades. We teased her by delivering a glass of water when she had clearly pointed to a picture of a sandwich, and Rosa would laugh and clunk her forehead with the palm of her gloved hand as if we exasperated her. Slowly, with thought, care and respect, we helped her to heal. And we didn't see Madame Durig again until after Rosa was discharged.

Maya, Victoria, Blythe, Pippa and I skied our hearts out in the Swiss Alps that season, and on the slopes we befriended a group of Australian skiers who were travelling the world by following the snow. Like Bambi at Selfridges, they talked of their homeland with pride. They made Australia sound enticingly warm, carefree and full of light and space and opportunity. As one Aussie said, 'Fifty million flies can't be wrong!' Amused by their laconic humour, and impressed that Australia was a hundred and eighty-six times the size of Switzerland, I was more than ever determined to visit the lucky country.

By the end of the snow season I had the atlas out and was ready to put the next part of my grand plan into action. Bermuda and Australia were both on my radar, but I had an important matter to settle before making a decision on either.

Did I want to carry on nursing?

CHAPTER 21

An Irresolute Tourist

Europe: Summer 1977

I WAS ENJOYING the work at Hôpital Sandoz but, truth be told, I was becoming a little bored. When I told my father this, he said, 'You've stopped learning, Maggie love. You need to be challenged.' But challenged by what? Another language? Another career? Not poverty again, surely.

I wrote to British universities requesting information on degree courses, to the Australian Embassy enquiring about a work visa, and posted another application to the King Edward VII Memorial Hospital in Bermuda. Picturing the secretary opening the letter, I could practically hear her saying, 'Oh, no, not her again!'

Victoria mentioned she had heard good things about Hôpital d'Aigle in the small historic town of Aigle at the eastern end of Lake Geneva, and one afternoon I drove along to investigate. In half an hour there was more action at Hôpital d'Aigle than I'd seen in a year at Sandoz. A helicopter arrived and nurses rushed around escorting a patient on a stretcher into the hospital. It was dramatic and exciting and I put Hôpital d'Aigle on my 'possibles' list.

The universities sent reams of information, all in

highfalutin education-speak that nobody who wasn't already at a university would understand. The Australian Embassy sent forms, which I completed and returned, and Bermuda offered me a nursing position, but I would have to take the job offer (i.e. carry on nursing) in order to live there. In Australia, once I had a work visa, I would hopefully be able to find any casual job on arrival. Everything went on my 'possibles' list for further consideration.

In April I was called to the Australian Embassy in London for an interview, which I thought strange for a simple work visa. I was also asked to send a photograph of myself and complete masses more forms.

The interview was unusual. The clerk looked at me, ticked a box, then asked me to sit down. I sat down. He pushed more forms across the desk and I signed them. Then I was told that if I was successful I would be notified in due course.

The explanation became clear in May when the Australian Embassy notified me that my permanent resident visa had been approved. Permanent resident visa? Unbelievably, I had signed up for the major prize.

Now, what to do? With too many choices, ideas about my future started thudding around in my brain, like wet towels in a tumble-dryer, and I was having trouble sleeping.

In June I left my *infirmière* position at Hôpital Sandoz and my much-loved apartment in Lausanne, deciding that a couple of months' driving around Europe with my friend Stella, who had leave, was the obvious tonic. It would hopefully recharge my batteries and help me to decide if I wanted to continue nursing.

It didn't. But with a clear head and renewed sense

of purpose, I decided to decline the position in Bermuda. I had already discarded Hôpital d'Aigle and the university idea. The simple truth was that I was so fortunate to receive an Australian resident's visa that it would be wrong not to use it. Who knew if I would pursue nursing when I got there? Did I even care?

I planned to be in England for a month, staying with my father and Aunt Joan in West Liss prior to flying out to Australia. That would give me an opportunity to visit friends in London and also see Richard and Esther, who were living not far away in Hythe, Hampshire. My brother was working at a hospital in Southampton and Esther was pregnant, which was very exciting news.

While I always relished visiting family, the real reason for the lengthy visit home was less fortuitous. A couple of weeks earlier, during a telephone call from Monte Carlo to my father, he had told me that Aunt Joan was 'quite unwell', a vague term from my father's medical lexicon that could mean anything from an infected splinter to raging anthrax. He sounded worried and I wanted to assess the situation for myself before gallivanting off to the other side of the world.

As soon as I saw Aunt Joan I knew things were serious. Pale and shaky, she was having trouble with her balance and speech. After greetings and a decent cup of tea, I traipsed across the field behind the house to where Joan's daughter, Suzie, lived. There I learned that my aunt had seen her local doctor and was to see a neurologist in early September. The neurologist, I knew, would order tests, which would take time, and then a treatment decision would be made, depending on the diagnosis.

Aunt Joan's illness terrified me. My greatest fear

was that she had a brain tumour and, like my mother (her first cousin), would die a dreadful death. I couldn't bear to lose another mother, and I couldn't imagine what losing another wife so soon would do to my father. More than anything, I didn't want Suzie to go through what I had experienced. I prayed the illness was something manageable, like Ménière's disease or late-onset migraine. Anything but cancer.

On my third day home my father's welcoming arms began to droop. The Johnsons (half of my genetic pool) must constantly be 'doing something', and even though I was looking after Aunt Joan (who had headaches and frequent dizzy spells) and cooking the meals, my father was displaying obvious displeasure at my other pursuits. It was apparent that snoozing on the sofa, soaking in a bubble bath and sunbathing on the back lawn were only options if the inactivity was accompanied by a book, a rousing Bach concerto in D minor or a challenging *Times* crossword.

Alert to impending advice that while I was sitting there I could mend a shirt, polish the silver or write to a relative no one had contacted in twenty-five years, I called the British Nursing Association and asked if they had any shifts available near West Liss. There was no point causing friction at home by looking idle, and I could do with the money: my bank account had taken a thorough beating on the continent.

'We've some night duty near you at a convent for old nuns,' advised an unenthusiastic female voice on the phone. 'The senior nurse nun is away and they need a state registered nurse to administer medications. You'd be working with nuns as well. To be honest, I'm having trouble finding someone to work there.'

Uncertain, I bit my lip. I'd been hoping for a few nights on a surgical ward at a local hospital. I hadn't worked in geriatrics for a while. Did I still have the patience needed to help the aged cope with their limitations? What about the back-breaking realities of lifting, transferring and turning patients? Hoists were not then in common use, and I hadn't lifted anything heavier than a gin and tonic in two months. And if I was already ambivalent about continuing my nursing career, geriatrics wasn't going to help matters.

Through the window I saw my father take a spade from the shed and march with horticultural intent towards the kitchen garden.

'Thank you,' I quickly told the woman on the phone. 'I'll take it.'

After telling me I had made her day, she rattled off the necessary details and I put down the receiver. Working in a convent with nuns who were caring for other nuns would be a first. I would have to put the handbrake on blasphemous exclamations, and having heard horror stories from convent schoolgirls, I was mildly fearful of knuckles or other Maggie parts receiving a wallop. Why, I wondered, was the nursing agency having trouble filling the position? Realizing I should have asked, I banished a developing frown and made a cup of tea for Aunt Joan.

Outside, I half expected to meet Beatrix Potter in the green and pleasant country garden. The sun was shining, blackbirds were chirping and bees were buzzing lazily around the honeysuckle that was holding up the old shed. My father was winding a wooden bucket of water up from the well.

Aunt Joan was sitting in a deckchair on the lawn

reading *Roots*, and Mathew, her West Highland white terrier, was digging up spring onions where my father had left the spade. The happy bucolic scene belied the undercurrent of angst.

I took Aunt Joan her tea, sat down on the grass beside her and chatted for a while until she fell asleep. Pulling the blanket over her knees, I retrieved her teacup and wandered over to the kitchen garden.

'I'm working a nursing shift later at a convent,' I told my father, and hastily added that I should rest beforehand. There was always a risk if an assistant was handy that it would be a perfect opportunity to spread compost on the garden.

Unusually nervous about a work assignment, I couldn't sleep and lay on my bed staring at the old black beams in the brick bedroom wall and the cabbage roses on the curtains. Later, after a cup of tea, I dressed in my nurse's uniform, pinned my King's badge to the collar and brushed my hair in a high ponytail. No make-up. No perfume. No offence.

'Don't swear and don't hit them back!' my father called as I drove off, which only served to increase my anxiety.

What had I let myself in for?

CHAPTER 22

A Lesson in Humility

Mount Alvernia, Hindhead, Surrey: August 1977

NESTLED IN HIGH-COUNTRY woodland near the Hampshire –
Surrey border, Mount Alvernia stood in as beautiful a
rural enclave as could be found anywhere in the British
Isles. A large Edwardian country home, it was a haven
where elderly nuns who had spent their lives nursing
the sick and poor could live out their final years being
cared for by other nuns, and occasionally, when a
medical situation required it, a state registered nurse
from an agency, which was where I came in.

It was a balmy evening and still light when I drove
through the lovely garden and pulled up in front of
Mount Alvernia. Pretty as a calendar picture, with ivy-
covered white walls and an abundance of small-paned
windows, the house had once been a hostel run by a
Mrs Bulley – 'a place where tired professional people
could breathe fine air and be saved from over-strain'. It
was renamed Mount Alvernia when the nuns took up
residence, after a hospital where they had worked.

A shortish, well-fed nun wearing a plain brown tunic
dress, muddy wellies and a shoulder-length veil was
standing near the front door. She was hosing a bed of

snapdragons and lupins, and occasionally splashing cobwebs off the window panes. Wishing with all my heart that I had never seen Fellini's Casanova erotically seducing a fake nun, I swallowed hard, repeated my newly learned mantra – 'Don't say "shit", don't say "Jesus", don't say "shit", don't say "Jesus"' – and duly climbed out of the car.

'They've sent us an angel,' the nun sang, and turned off the water. As I blushed with embarrassment, she struggled to re-coil the reluctant hose into a large pot. Putting down my bag, I went to help.

'You have a beautiful garden,' I said, initiating social niceties.

'It is now,' she replied stoically, 'but you should have seen the mess when the good Lord was doing it himself.'

It was an old gag that I'd heard before, but I laughed and her chubby face lit up. It was obviously a favourite joke, and she appreciated a receptive audience.

'I'll be Sister Eugenia,' she said, and before I could say my own name, she quickly added, 'Come in, will you, come in to the house and have yourself a pot of tea and a scone. Sister Flora has some of her strawberry jam waiting.'

So far so good, I thought. No wallops. No stake through the heart.

Looping her arm through mine, Sister Eugenia led me towards the house. Once inside she pulled off the wellies, brushed off her dress and eased her feet into sturdy black thick-soled shoes. Silently I followed her into a spacious old-fashioned kitchen where I was introduced to Sister Mary Agatha and Sister Flora.

Like Sister Eugenia, they appeared to be in their

mid to late forties and were dressed in similar brown knee-length dresses and short veils. Sister Mary Agatha was tall and willowy and at first glance I thought she was wearing a party nose with plastic glasses attached. Further inspection revealed an unfortunate beaky-shaped appendage and horn-rimmed glasses with thick lenses. She looked like a cross between Groucho Marx and a vision-impaired spoonbill. In contrast, Sister Flora was medium-sized in every way, with warm brown eyes nestled in a pretty face. They were not wearing wimples and I could see they each had short, serviceable haircuts to which they'd attached their veils.

'I'm Sister Johnson,' I said, and quickly realized the potential for misunderstanding. 'I mean, I'm a qualified nurse, not one of . . . not a nun or anything religious.'

'We know,' Sister Flora said with a hint of amusement, her brown eyes glowing. 'Do you have a first name?'

I nodded. They didn't look like the haircloth penitents I had anticipated, although the power of authority bestowed on them by their dress and distinctive veils was unnerving.

'And what will that be?' Sister Eugenia coaxed.

'Oh, Margaret – Maggie,' I said.

Sister Mary Agatha smiled and pulled out a wheel-back chair at the kitchen table. 'Then sit down, Sister Maggie, and we'll tell you about our dear sisters.' Her voice was soft and her words flowed smooth like warm honey.

Irish, and with smiles as wide as four-lane highways, the three of them fussed around preparing refreshments in the old kitchen. Watching, I noticed they all limped and each had an unfortunate foot deformity that had necessitated alterations to their sturdy black shoes. In Mary Agatha's case, there was also a calliper on her left calf. I found myself wondering if, in their younger years when girls from large Irish families were expected to marry, it was decided that the damage would dash any hopes of love, marriage and children, and Eugenia, Mary Agatha and Flora had instead been steered towards vows of poverty, chastity and obedience. I hoped not.

Over tea and scones from mismatched china, I learned we were caring for about twenty elderly resident nuns, or 'dear sisters', as Sister Mary Agatha referred to them. Hailing from all corners of the British Isles, most were frail from advanced age, a few had dementia, two were convalescing after surgery for fractured neck of femur, one had shingles, another a recurrence of malaria, and yet another was recuperating from a total hip replacement.

'D'you have any questions?' Sister Flora asked me, her eyebrows raised in expectation. 'About anything?'

I had a few, mainly about the nun business.

Between them, and this is entirely my take on their explanations, the sisters told me there were many religious orders but only two types of nun – sisters who lived in the world and devoted their lives to God's merciful works, such as nursing, teaching, and caring for the poor and destitute, and others who were ascetics and lived apart from the world in closed convents and prayed to God for the world.

'And the sisters who live here?' I asked.

'Our dear sisters have spent their lives nursing the sick, at home and in far corners of the world,' Sister Mary Agatha said.

A Lesson in Humility

That accounted for the malaria case. There is a certain strain that can recur years later, and the fevers and chills are frightful. I knew this first hand as my father had suffered from occasional recurrences of the malaria that he had contracted in Africa when he was a young merchant seaman. It was one of the few times he admitted defeat and took to his bed during the day without a book or a crossword.

Curious as to why the nuns weren't wearing long black habits, and taking care not to make it sound like an accusation, I asked cautiously, 'Why do you wear . . . brown dresses?'

There was an awkward silence. Then Sister Flora frowned and looked down at the dowdy knee-length dress she was wearing. 'This old thing!' she said, and we all laughed. It was a timely ice-breaker and Flora went on to explain that traditional habits were not functional at Mount Alvernia. As I was to learn, in addition to nursing duties, the women did everything from mowing the lawns to repairing the roof.

Our tea party over, Sister Mary Agatha gave me a whirlwind tour of the rambling house and its many bedrooms, utility rooms and cupboards, or 'presses' as she called them. Limping from room to room, she introduced me to the elderly nuns so that I could match a diagnosis with the correct dear sister. As they all looked the same to me – frail elderly women with short, wispy grey hair, cream nightgowns, grey shawls and ready smiles for anyone who entered their room – matching a dear sister with her diagnosis and her room would be a problem, particularly if they all got up and moved around.

Once I had my bearings, or thought I had, we set

to work – bedtime drinks (which for some, instead of night sedation, meant a glass of pale ale or Guinness, a drink they referred to as 'the black stuff'), calamine lotion on shingles sores (which they referred to as 'the pink stuff'), a drug round, which was the reason that my professional services were required, tepid sponging for the poor soul with malaria fever, general help with cleaning teeth, painfully slow walking trips to and from the bathroom, refilling hot water bottles (no electric blankets), and preparing those who were physically able to attend the night-time prayers observed by the nuns. Thankfully, most of the dear sisters were small so heavy lifting wasn't an issue.

I was lost several times on the first night, disorientated by corridors that had no identifiable landmarks, and could have done with a few well-placed Val Doonican posters. Surprisingly, the bedrooms, when I found them, were comfortable and cosy with colourful knitted patchwork covers on the simple wrought-iron beds. Glass jam-jars of fresh roses adorned plain, Shaker-style bedside tables and, as I'd expected, simple holy items hung on the walls.

Intent on visiting a dear sister with dementia, I opened a door and found Sister Eugenia sitting on the bed with her legs up and her large motherly arm cradling a tiny elderly lady. Eugenia was reading *Noddy Goes to the Seaside* and pointing at the pictures. Looking up and seeing my delighted expression, she winked at me and said, 'It's Sister Endellion's favourite book. She loves the part where the crab gets Noddy's toe.'

Leaving them to it, I quietly closed the door. As an experienced agency nurse, I could tell when good care had been consistent, and while it might seem an inappropriate phrase, at Mount Alvernia the devil was most definitely in the detail. There was no pervading smell of urine that you often find in nursing homes, and not a bedsore in the place. Finger- and toenails were well trimmed, ears were clean, false teeth fitted mouths, hearing aids had batteries, spectacles were clean and labelled, residents were well-nourished and well-hydrated (a sign that patience was taken with meals and drinks) and handbells and Bibles were within arm's reach. It was good to see elderly women who had devoted their lives to others receiving the best nursing care in their own dotage.

Throughout the night I had to keep reminding myself that I was the senior nurse and therefore in charge. I was feeling a bit outclassed and leadership wasn't happening naturally, but my workmates rather sweetly went out of their way to ask questions that implied my authority – 'What is this drug for, Sister Maggie?'; 'Would you come and look at this dressing and advise us on further treatment, Sister Maggie?'; 'Do you think we could give Sister Marguerite a wee glass of the black stuff, Sister Maggie?' I was certain they already knew the answers.

After settling our charges, I was hoping for another bash at Flora's scones, but it wasn't to be. In the kitchen, Sister Eugenia abruptly ordered me to stoke the boiler and forced a brass coal scuttle and a torch into my hands. And she wasn't smiling.

'What?' I exclaimed, startled by her demand.

'The coal shed's outside,' she said sharply.

I stared at her. Then I looked at Flora and Mary Agatha who were busying themselves with washing up at the sink, seemingly oblivious to my plight.

Maybe this was some sort of test.

The nuns weren't to know, but I was used to stoking boilers from my childhood. I had loathed the job then, and I wasn't impressed at being asked, as a state registered nurse, to do it now.

As if sensing my bewilderment, Sister Flora turned around and explained, 'It's penance, to be sure, Sister Maggie.'

'What the ... What for?' I spluttered, unable to hide my indignation.

'For settling Sister Sarah in Sister Gertrude's bed and vice versa,' Sister Mary Agatha sang in her honeyed voice.

Sister Eugenia looked stern, Sister Mary Agatha looked guilty, and the edges of Sister Flora's mouth were twitching. Whatever this was, they were all in on it.

Since my early days of agency nursing I had found it best to have as low an impact as possible on a new work environment. I had discovered that the important thing was to watch and learn from nurses already there, and to pitch in with the heavy work. Nobody likes a snotty cow who marches in and starts throwing her weight around.

I narrowed my eyes and looked at each of them. If they expected me to refuse to stoke the boiler, or ask how to do it, they had another think coming. I took a deep breath and headed outside. So much for being in charge.

The boiler at Mount Alvernia stood in the corner of the kitchen and was fuelled by anthracite. Year round it heated the hot water, and in winter I suppose it took care of the heating. When I had finished shovelling anthracite into the scuttle I lugged it back to the kitchen, easily opened the boiler and tipped a load inside. Then I poked it around a bit before closing it and topping up the Aga stove as well. Secretly, I think all three nuns were impressed. I know I was.

The incident was not spoken of again and normal pleasant communications were resumed. At two o'clock Sisters Eugenia and Mary Agatha retired to bed. Sister Flora was to wake them in the morning unless we needed help earlier. Sister Flora, I learned, would go to bed at eight, after breakfast.

Stunned, I hadn't realized the sisters had no defined work hours. I'd assumed other staff would appear in the morning. I was humbled to learn that the three women lived and worked at Mount Alvernia, slept when they could and, apart from religious devotion, their whole life revolved around caring for the dear sisters, the house and the grounds.

As soon as the other two had gone to bed, Sister Flora, who I had already guessed was more relaxed than the others, turned on the radio, then scrubbed her hands as though she were about to perform surgery. I did the same. When in Rome . . .

'Green beans first,' she said, and dried her hands on a heavily frayed tea towel that had probably seen service in the Crimea.

Listening to pop songs on Radio 1, over successive nights after the others had retired, Flora and I topped, tailed and stringed pounds of freshly picked green beans, prepared and kneaded dough, peeled and stewed sweet Cox's orange pippins that Eugenia had picked in the morning, darned ancient threadbare habits, mended substantial-looking undergarments on an old Singer treadle sewing machine, glued rubber soles to black orthopaedic shoes, scrubbed pine tables, ground cold roast lamb in a metal hand-mincer for the world's largest shepherd's pie, read from *A Passage to India* to a dear sister who couldn't sleep and had spent her working life with the poor in Calcutta, cast stitches of navy wool on to large needles for hot-water-bottle covers and blanket squares, scattered nuts and stale bread outside for the skylarks and squirrels, and cooked vats of porridge that would have fed the Royal Navy in Gibraltar. In between chores, Flora and I made rounds of the bedrooms, turned frail dear sisters where and when required to prevent bedsores, and attended to other personal needs.

And you know what? I loved it. I absolutely loved it. The satisfaction of being nurse, cook, baker, seamstress, reader, cleaner, boot-maker and boiler-stoker was like nothing I had experienced before. I might have had a bee in my bonnet that first night over Eugenia's request for me to stoke the boiler (which, as a matter of pride, I continued to attend to without being asked), but it was the anticipated pleasure of the work ahead and the chance to spend more time with Eugenia, Mary Agatha and Flora that easily had me returning to Mount Alvernia.

I enjoyed the job so much that the only time I took off was for my friend Pippa's wedding to her Swiss doctor boyfriend, Gilbert. Other friends, including Maya and her fiancé, Maurice, had come over from Switzerland to England and, in the haste of fitting everything in, I had forgotten to remove my red nail polish before returning to Mount Alvernia. If they disapproved, Sisters Eugenia and Mary Agatha said nothing, but I quickly realized that Sister Flora was fascinated by my nails. More than once I caught her covertly examining her own splayed fingers.

A Lesson in Humility

That night, after Eugenia and Mary Agatha had retired to bed and our nursing chores were done, Sister Flora and I set about stewing and bottling apples for winter. As we stood at the large sink and peeled and sliced pounds of Keswick Codlins, Flora asked me about the wedding. She wanted to know everything about Pippa's dress and hair, the flowers and the wedding cake. Surprised by her keen interest in what she must surely consider frivolous matters, I told her about our beautiful fairy queen, Pippa, and how, even when not getting married, she always wore feminine Laura Ashley dresses and often carried a parasol and a basket.

It crossed my mind that pretty Flora might be suffering pangs of regret that she would never enjoy such a day herself, so I told her that I wasn't much of a one for wedding frou-frou and that if I ever got married it would be a simple affair. I sensed that she didn't believe me, but it was the truth.

We tipped the Codlins into two big stock pots on the Aga, heaped in sugar and a little water, then added cinnamon sticks to one pan and cloves to the other. Sitting down to write labels for the jars, I noticed Flora frowning. Worried I had offended her in some way, I asked, 'Is anything wrong?'

She shook her head. 'It's nothing.'

Something was definitely wrong.

'Come on,' I said encouragingly. 'Tell me, Flora, please.' By now we had dispensed with formalities when we were alone.

Flora suddenly plonked her hands flat on the table and in a hurried voice, as though if she didn't say it now she never would, she blurted out, 'Do you think . . . I mean . . . could you paint my nails for me, Maggie?'

Touched that she had asked me, I couldn't hide my pleasure. 'I'd love to, Flora,' I said happily. 'We'll do it tomorrow when the others have gone to bed.'

Taking a big breath, Flora grinned in mock conspiracy and pointed at my red fingernails. 'That red colour, too.'

The next night, when everyone had gone to bed we made hot chocolate, turned on the radio and sat down next to each other at the kitchen table.

'Are you ready?' Flora asked excitedly.

'Uh-huh.'

'Then let's begin,' she said, and elaborately placed her hands on the table as if she were about to perform a Chopin piano concerto.

Not yet chronologically old, Flora's hands had the appearance of a woman twenty years her senior, and I knew the rough skin and calluses had been earned the hard way. Privately I felt uncomfortable desecrating such evidence of good works with frivolous splodges of something called 'Starlet Scarlet', but I had promised Flora I would do it.

For dramatic effect I vigorously shook the bottle of nail polish, undid it and extracted the brush, carefully wiping a little off on the rim of the bottle. Pausing, I looked up at Flora who, eyes big as saucers, was fixated on her nails.

'Are you sure you want me to do this?' I asked, hoping she would abandon the idea.

'Oh, just do it, will you?' she gushed, and it took me some time to stop laughing enough to steady my hand.

When I had finished, Flora examined her nails and giggled with delight. 'Aww . . .' she trilled. 'They're fine. Thank you, Maggie.'

288

A Lesson in Humility

'Don't do anything for ten minutes so they dry,' I said, and she left her hands on the table out of harm's way. Right where she could see them.

Suddenly the song playing on the radio stopped and a man's voice advised that the broadcast was interrupted to make a serious announcement: Elvis Aaron Presley, aged forty-two, had been found dead at Graceland, his mansion in Memphis, Tennessee.

Speechless, I couldn't believe my ears.

Flora bowed her head and crossed herself, careful not to catch her nails. I think she said a prayer.

'I loved Elvis,' I said sadly. And I had. I had seen every Elvis film, purchased every record and scratched his name inside a heart on my pre-war wooden desk at school.

We observed a long respectful silence until Flora leaned across the table towards me. 'Can I move now, d'you think?' she said, in a hushed tone.

'In a minute,' I told her. 'Can I ask you a question first?'

'You can.' She looked up at me in anticipation, her brown eyes dancing.

I paused, thinking how to word my thoughts. The resident state registered nurse, Sister Bernadette, would be returning from Ireland in the morning and, as this was my last night duty at Mount Alvernia, I wanted to ask Flora about something that was bothering me.

Hoping she would be honest, I said, 'Well, the agency told me they were having trouble finding an SRN to work here. Why was that, do you think?'

In response, Flora threw back her head and let out a loud hoot. 'You should have seen your face when

Sister Eugenia told you to stoke the boiler. You were a picture. Everyone else has refused and never come back!'

Relieved, I smiled at Flora who, to my mind, had rather speedily dispensed with polite homage to Elvis. 'So, it *was* some sort of test?' I said.

Flora nodded. 'Aye, it was. It amuses Sister Eugenia. She likes to measure the mettle of agency nurses . . . Says it sorts out the racehorses from the donkeys.'

'Racehorses and donkeys?' I questioned.

'Aye, we don't want any donkeys here. Anyway, you're a racehorse and you passed with flying colours, to be sure. I thought Sister Eugenia was going to kiss you when you filled the stove as well. And then when you kept on doing it, we couldn't believe it.'

'Good grief,' I said quietly. Trickster nuns. Who'd have thought?

Later, after Flora had experimented with holding teacups in a queenly manner, and elegantly draping her fingers over the arms of chairs in the sitting room, I took off the nail polish with varnish remover, hid the evidence in my car and we prepared for the morning arrival of the other sisters.

In honour of my last shift at Mount Alvernia, and as soon as the dear sisters had finished their breakfast, we nurses sat down at the kitchen table to eat porridge with warm milk and Demerara sugar, followed by toast with lashings of butter and Flora's strawberry jam.

'You know, there's a funny chemical smell in here,' Sister Eugenia remarked, screwing up her nose and sniffing around.

And indeed there was. Even though I had opened the windows and the back door, the smell of nail-varnish remover still hung in the air. Flora cast me an anxious look.

'I expect it's something the highly qualified nursing sister put in the boiler that she was told to stoke,' I said calmly, raising my brows and widening my eyes at Sister Eugenia as if to say 'I'm wise to your trickery.'

At first, Sister Eugenia looked confused, but then a wicked grin settled across her wise and weathered face. Slowly she raised her teacup to me. It was, I felt, an apology of sorts, and quite possibly the best I was going to get.

As I drove away from Mount Alvernia on that final morning, I knew I had experienced something very special. And that I would miss those thoughtful, generous, complicated women. The unexpected business with the boiler had confirmed to me that swallowing my professional pride, saying nothing, and just getting on with a job was the best way to garner respect from work colleagues. It was a valuable lesson in humility and, unbeknown to the sisters, they had also rekindled my nursing mojo. I was now certain that, in one form or another, I was going to carry on nursing. In Australia.

CHAPTER 23

An Interlude with an
American Legend

King Edward VII Hospital, West Sussex, Midhurst:
September 1977

IT WAS EARLY September and I was packing my trunk for
shipment to Australia when Aunt Joan was diagnosed
with a brain tumour. How could this be happening to
my mother's first cousin, and at a similar age?

Aunt Joan underwent surgery and was given
her chance of survival in percentages, which we
understood to mean that nobody knew how long she
would live. She came home to convalesce and prepare
for follow-up treatment. 'Your father, Suzie and I can
cope with this,' she told me. 'You must go to Australia
as planned.'

I was in a quandary. I felt guilty about leaving, but
also that I might be in the way if I stayed. I knew that
Suzie was an emotionally strong and capable woman,
and that my father could cook and clean and look after
his wife. After all, the poor man had done it before.

'You are not indispensable!' Aunt Joan insisted,

292

when I whined once too often about leaving, and so it was settled. I was going to Australia.

Even so, I dragged my heels over buying a plane ticket until Richard found insurance that funded my trip home in a family emergency. I bought a ticket and insurance and called the nursing agency for a few days' work to replenish my bank account.

'We have a week on the private wing at King Edward VII Hospital in Midhurst,' the woman said. 'Nursing an elderly American lady.'

'Is she infectious?' I asked, thinking of Joan.

'No.'

'So what's wrong with her?' I pressed.

'She's American,' the woman said, and I wasn't sure if I was supposed to laugh, so I didn't.

'I'll take it,' I said, thinking that if I wasn't going to King Edward VII in Bermuda, I might as well work at King Edward VII in Midhurst.

Set in the beautiful West Sussex countryside, the King Edward VII started life as a sanatorium and was converted to a hospital in the sixties. These days, it has been turned into luxury apartments, but it was still in the hospital phase when I rolled up the driveway as a private nurse to look after 'the American lady'.

She's probably the size of a London bus, I thought uncharitably, as I opened the door to her room, but I was wrong. My first impression was of a fairy peeking out from an enormous display of brightly coloured flowers. Further inspection revealed a petite woman of mature years sitting on the bed with her legs over the side. She was trying to stand up without knocking over the flower vases on the bed-table.

'Oh dear, it's like a cottage garden in here,' she

mused, her accent soft and sweet. She looked younger than her years and had the face of a porcelain doll. I guessed she had been rather a beauty in her youth.

'Here, let me help,' I offered.

'Can we walk?' she asked, once standing.

'Just a short distance,' I said. 'If it goes well, we can do more tomorrow.'

'What is your name?' she asked.

'Maggie,' I said. At full height she didn't reach my shoulder. I felt like a carthorse next to a gazelle as we took baby steps across the room.

'I shall call you Margaret,' she said, sounding determined.

'Actually, it's Maggie,' I corrected.

She stopped walking and looked at me. 'I prefer Margaret.'

Straight away I knew my place. Boundaries were set.

We walked a little further before I helped her back to bed.

'Are you in a good mood, Margaret?' she asked.

'Yes,' I answered. 'Why?'

Passing a silver hairbrush to me, she said, 'Because I never let anyone brush my hair if they are cross.'

With some effort, she eased her legs over the side of the bed again so I could let down her hair from behind.

Unpinning her French roll, I let the fine silver-grey hair fall down her back, so long it would easily have reached her knees.

'Beautiful hair,' I mumbled, as I gently brushed.

'It used to be, Margaret,' she said with regret.

We were silent for a while until she said, in an authoritative tone, 'When we have finished my hair you shall be the nurse and I will be your obedient patient.'

'All right,' I said, and we smiled at each other.

Throughout the week, we retained our roles – for nursing matters I was in charge, and for everything else, I wasn't. The health of my American lady improved quickly, which surprised and delighted me. I had seen this sort of resilience before – slight women whose frail appearance belied an inner physical strength, and my American lady, while remaining feminine and gracious, was titanium wrapped in pink tissue paper.

After my fifth day at the hospital, I was telling my father and Joan at dinner about my quirky little American lady.

'What's her name?' Aunt Joan asked.

'I call her Miss Gish,' I said. 'I'm not allowed to call her Lillian.'

'Lillian Gish!' Aunt Joan exclaimed.

My father also looked astonished. 'You mean you are looking after Lillian Gish and you don't know who she is?'

I shook my head. 'No idea, but she receives a lot of flowers.'

Both Aunt Joan and my father started laughing, and if nothing else it was good to see Aunt Joan amused.

Miss Gish, it appeared, was famous. Rarely off the stage or screen in the early twentieth century, she was a silent movie star and favourite leading lady of the American movie mogul Mr D. W. Griffith. Known as the First Lady of American Cinema, the American Film Institute had named her the seventeenth greatest female star of all time, and I had named her the American Lady in Room Fourteen.

My father was still laughing about it when, the following day, we drove to Southampton docks to ship my trunk out to Australia. Safe inside, wrapped in clothes, were Eddie Bear, my teapots, sherry glasses and the porcelain umbrella stand.

CHAPTER 24

Wild Colonial Girl

Sydney, Australia: October 1977

'How do I know your plane arrived from England?' the Australian Customs officer asked me. He looked about fourteen and had sandy hair and freckles everywhere, even on his hands.

'Because it says so on my ticket,' I replied.

'Nope,' he said, and grinned stupidly. 'It's because the whining didn't stop when they turned off the engines.'

I smiled benignly and pictured my umbrella jammed in his left ear. Such was my introduction to the lucky country and Pommy jokes.

Establishing myself in Sydney proved to be much easier than I'd expected, and within a short timeframe I had rented a reasonably priced room in a shared house in the harbour suburb of Mosman, discovered a great pub called the Oaks Hotel, registered with the Nurses Registration Board and secured a job interview.

Amazed at how smoothly things were going, I leaned against the outside wall of Sydney Opera House and took stock. I had traded a soggy grey London autumn for a glorious spring day in Sydney, and I'd just been interviewed and accepted a registered nurse (RN) position on a general surgical ward at Sydney Hospital – a grand-looking sandstone establishment a short walk from where I was standing. If I passed the medical, I would start work in two weeks. It was all too good to be true.

In front of me Sydney Harbour Bridge cast shimmering shadows on the sparkling water as ferries chugged back and forth between Circular Quay and the harbour suburbs. For a moment I took delight in the fact that it was I, the wilful younger child of the Johnsons, who'd made it to Australia, not my much smarter brother with his dreams of being a flying doctor in the outback. Then I remembered that Richard had been refused a visa because of recurring health problems following his toboggan accident, and I felt terribly guilty. For about two minutes.

My father had sailed twice to Melbourne, but never Sydney, and I wished he was with me, seeing what I was seeing. Smiling, I thought of how he had told me quite seriously that the volume of water in Sydney Harbour was a unit of measurement known as a Sydharb, and that it would show I was intelligent with a wide range of interests if I could somehow work this little-known fact into conversations.

Last, I thought of my mother and the day we had sat on her bed and watched the Queen open Sydney Opera House. I placed my hands on the wall either side of me for a deeper connection with the building. It was four years since Mum had died, but it still felt like yesterday. I was momentarily overwhelmed, and tears flooded my eyes.

Wild Colonial Girl

Brushing them away, I set off for Circular Quay to catch the ferry to Mosman Bay. I had two weeks to familiarize myself with the subliminal knowledge of a new life in a new country – where to buy decent bread and vegetables, how different cuts of meat were defined, where to catch a bus into the city, a bank that didn't view women as liabilities – the basics that formed the small building blocks of a bigger life.

Those two weeks were a voyage of discovery – the heady scent of tropical flowers at dusk, the raucous screech of brightly coloured parrots, men in safari suits and knee-length socks, distances measured in time instead of length, suburbs called Woolloomooloo and Kirribilli, tradesmen trucks with dogs and surfboards in the back, pubs called 'hotels' and an afternoon called an 'arvo' – and all of it dressed in brilliant sunshine.

I'd been in Sydney a few days when I joined new friends for a swim at Obelisk Beach, a small sandy cove in the harbour with steep hillsides that necessitated patient negotiation to climb safely down. It was also one of Sydney's nudist beaches and in those days frequented mostly by families. I'd harboured a desire to swim in the buff since I was a young child, an impulse to be blamed entirely on saggy, home-made swimsuits. At twenty-five, I owned a non-saggy bikini, but I still yearned to swim naked in the sea. And as no one really knew me in Australia, and as the beach was secluded, I considered it as good a time as any to give my grown-up body and its added attractions a nudie swim.

So in I went, and it was a thrilling kind of freedom, although a little scary because I didn't know what was swimming beneath me. In another sense it instilled in me a profound feeling of being part of nature and my insignificant place in the big picture.

There were luxury motor cruisers anchored offshore, their passengers peeling off clothes and throwing themselves over the side with abandon. I had the clever idea to limit exposure back to my towel by immersing myself in a group who had swum ashore, but my plan was thwarted. A trimaran that had pulled down its sails was drifting perilously towards an anchored motor cruiser. A handsome-looking man standing on the bow of the trimaran was waving for attention.

'We've lost power. Can someone fend off?' he called casually, surprisingly calm considering what was about to happen. Having already inveigled myself among the group, I had no choice but to join them, swim out to deeper water and help nudge the stricken yacht out of harm's way until it slowly cruised to a halt.

'Thanks,' the man said. He was grinning mischievously.

Treading water, I watched, fascinated, as the man effortlessly dropped a heavy anchor over the side. He was tall with an athletic build and a golden tan, and his sun-bleached hair was wavy and worn just a shade too long for a city worker. I guessed he was a country boy.

As if sensing my inspection, the man looked straight at me.

'Hello, you,' he said, and in among the gym-box packaging I saw gravity and shyness in his blue-grey eyes.

And that was how I met my husband, Jay.

Wild Colonial Girl

American and nine years older than me, Jay moved into my life with a teaching degree, a tennis racket, a set of golf clubs, a half-share in a yacht and a lot of good friends. Fearless and with nerves of steel, he was the first man I'd ever met who had no need to impress, no wish to be important, and no desire for possessions unless you could play sport with them. A little shy, he was genuinely interested in other people, and he was kind, thoughtful and very, very funny. He was, in every respect, his own man. And mine, of course.

Deemed healthy by the man conducting pre-employment medicals at Sydney Hospital, I attended lectures on the hospital's policies and procedures, emergency evacuation, health and safety regulations, et cetera, et cetera. All boxes ticked, I started work on the ward, and it was immediately apparent that every patient had kidney disease, many on dialysis. Somehow I was on a renal ward, not a general surgical ward as had been agreed. Politely, I informed the ward sister of the mistake.

'You must have agreed to this ward,' she remarked, surprise in her voice.

'No, I didn't,' I assured her. A feeling of unease swept over me as I left her to sort it out.

I hadn't looked after renal patients in years, and since then there had been a great deal of progress in treatments, dialysis and transplants. To say I was uncomfortable on the ward was an understatement.

An experienced nurse can walk on to any ward and see at a glance what needs to be done – which intravenous infusion requires changing, who is looking boss-eyed because they are desperate to use the bathroom, who is chilly and could use a blanket, who is falling asleep in a chair and should be returned to bed, and who is in pain and in need of medication – and I kept busy doing these general things until a doctor asked me to clear a blockage in a patient's shunt.

Embarrassed that I had no idea how to do that, which didn't instil confidence in the doctor or the patient, I asked another RN to show me how. She showed me, but the message from her was clear: if I didn't know what I was doing on that busy ward, I was putting patients' lives at risk. In agreement, I returned to the ward sister, who advised me that she'd been told I would not be moved.

I worked another early duty, making sure never to do anything without asking for supervision, a situation that drove everyone nuts and caused a backlog of work. Then came my first late duty, starting at 2.30 p.m. and finishing at 11 p.m. Unfortunately there was no public transport to Mosman after 11 p.m., so I waited for a taxi, which cost an arm and a leg, and fell into bed after midnight. Then I had to get up at 5.30 a.m. with the sparrows to start an early duty at 7 a.m. the next day.

It was only by nurses standing up to unprofessional treatment from employers that change could be effected, and I resigned the following afternoon, disillusioned that my first foray into Australian nursing had been such a disaster. I'd anticipated that Australian hospitals would be ahead of Europe in their treatment of nurses but, sadly, in 1977 things were still in the dark ages.

It wasn't too hard to figure out that low staffing

levels and poor conditions were a contributing factor to the desperate shortage of trained nurses in Australia (an opinion based on no research whatsoever), and why so many Aussie nurses had left to work in Britain. Australian nurses were already fighting for improved conditions and pay with marches, pickets, lobbying of ministers, rallies and strikes. Without knowing it, and having sustained only minor injury, I had walked into a war zone.

Realizing that if I was going to nurse in Australia it would have to be outside the hospital system, I wrote letters seeking industrial nursing positions, posted some to factories and handed others in at city department stores and Sydney Opera House. The only response was from someone at Sydney Opera House who advised they would contact me if a nursing position became available in the future.

Finding another job wasn't going to be easy. Perhaps I'd been too hasty in resigning from Sydney Hospital.

Jay and I talked of travelling the world and meeting each other's families. The end of an Australian autumn seemed like a good time to purchase round-the-world tickets and pack our bags.

As permanent Australian residents, we could retain that privilege only if we returned to Australia within three years of leaving, but we had no plans to return. Who knew where we would end up living?

It was early June when we island-hopped through the Pacific and travelled across America to Jay's hometown in upstate New York. There I promptly fell in love with Hershey chocolate, buffalo wings, beef on kimmelweck rolls and Jay's relatives. Dragging me away from his mother's cooking wasn't easy, but by high summer we had arrived in England to visit my family and meet the newest Johnson, my brother's son Ben.

All excitement was dashed when I saw Aunt Joan. She was extremely unwell and the cancer, as it had with my mother, was claiming her life at a premature age. I rolled up my sleeves to pitch in but was made to roll them down again. I wasn't needed. My father and Suzie were coping as well as anyone copes in such a situation. Besides, Aunt Joan was unsettled by my presence in the house, confused at times as to who Jay and I were.

I had a strong feeling that I didn't belong in this part of my family any more, and that I was, as I had so often been in my younger years after Richard's accident, in the way a bit. Rather than upset the household, Jay and I went down to Hythe on the south coast and stayed with Richard, Esther and baby Ben, who was already eight months old. We had a lovely few days together before Jay and I flew to Switzerland for the winter.

It was only a short flight back to England if I was needed, and neither Jay nor I wanted to spend a bleak winter in England. Much better to have usable cold weather for snow sports, and I was sure we would both find work in Switzerland. After all, I had terrific references from the hospitals in Lausanne, particularly the ones I'd written myself.

CHAPTER 25

Get Ready, Get Set, Snow!

Hôpital d'Aigle, Switzerland: 1978–9

IT WAS A glorious day when we arrived at Villars in the Swiss Alps. Wildflowers dotted the lush green hillsides and scarlet geraniums spilled from window boxes on picture-perfect chalets. The views of snow-capped mountains in the Dents-du-Midi and Mont Blanc massif were spectacular and Jay couldn't stop smiling.

By now, Victoria and Blythe were nursing at Hôpital d'Aigle, the hospital that had been on my 'possibles' list when I'd left Sandoz. Blythe had already canvassed a nursing position for me, and the day after we arrived I was sitting in an office at Hôpital d'Aigle, waiting while the head nurse examined my credentials. Idly I wondered if anything exciting had happened in Switzerland while I'd been away – a criminal speaking rudely to a policeman perhaps, or the train from Paris arriving four minutes late.

'Everything is in order,' the head nurse proclaimed, as he handed back my passport and work permit. 'We need experienced nurses who speak French on the surgical floor.'

I tensed, instantly recalling the disastrous surgical

ward allocation in Sydney. 'What sort of surgery?' I asked, trying not to sound as though I'd been responsible for the deaths of thousands of patients following a particular type of operation.

'A bit of everything,' he said, spreading his arms wide. 'Stomach, gall bladder and small-bowel surgery, hernia repair, some vascular and orthopaedic, and trauma that arrives by helicopter.'

It sounded just what I wanted. We agreed that I would start in a week and he stood up, my cue to leave.

By the following day Jay had arranged to pick apples in the nearby Rhône Valley and had also lined up work on the ski slopes for when the snow arrived in a few months' time. Nobody mentioned that Jay couldn't ski. Or speak French.

From the minute I started nursing on the busy surgical floor at Hôpital d'Aigle, I loved it. Many nurses had worked there for years, a sure sign that nurse–patient ratios were good and everyone was happy.

The senior qualified nurse on my floor was a highly experienced live wire from Chile, and the rest of us were registered nurses with a range of extra certificates from other European countries and Canada – and there is no doubt that both nurses and patients benefited from our diverse backgrounds and our different ways of approaching patient care. Although French was our common language, we had a mishmash of accents to entertain our patients. Swiss-French nurses from Canton Vaud spoke the slow, languid rhythm of Vaudoise, I had the apparently hilarious plummy diction of the British, the French-Canadians offered the strange but attractive Québécois, the

Swiss-Germans murdered French vowels with their guttural sounds, and our illustrious Chilean leader had the delightful Spanish lisp thing going on.

My own French rapidly came up to speed, but some of it was an affront to French grammar. Herr Yoder, a Swiss-German patient who spoke fluent French, often told me so. Aged seventy, he had an air of past importance and was not happy that he had fractured his pelvis and was confined to bed. And he was furious that he was being nursed by infants.

The infants in question were myself and Manon, the younger of our two French-Canadian nurses. Light and lithe as a dancer, Manon worked as quickly as she talked, which was much of the time. Endlessly fascinated by English expressions, she used them whenever the opportunity presented itself.

One morning Manon and I were prepping a patient for theatre when Herr Yoder buzzed frantically for the umpteenth time. 'By gollies and Joves,' Manon said, exasperated.

'I'll go,' I said.

Entering Herr Yoder's room, I noticed a pained expression on his face. '*Mes bijoux de famille sont mal mis,*' he complained.

Processing a quick translation, I assumed important jewellery was badly placed. Probably his watch. It would only take a second to look for it, so I quickly checked under the bed, behind the pillows, then lifted the duvet and searched the bedding. While I did this, Herr Yoder had the sort of expression on his face that people have when they are utterly amazed by what they are seeing.

'I'll return in a minute and have a proper look,' I said, and left the room.

No sooner was I back with Manon than Herr Yoder started yelling and buzzing again for assistance.

Manon said she would give him a piece of her brain and left the room.

Five minutes later I found Manon outside Herr Yoder's room, slumped to the floor and helpless with laughter.

'What is it?' I begged. 'What's happened?'

'Oh, cheeses,' she said, and reverting to her native tongue managed to tell me that the poor devil was sitting on his testicles and extremely uncomfortable. 'And you were looking for them!' Tears of laughter ran down her cheeks.

I gasped in horror. Of course. *Bijoux de famille*. Family jewels!

From then on, Herr Yoder delighted in telling anyone who'd listen that I was far too young and inexperienced to be a nurse. It goes without saying that a few doctors offered to show me the location of their own testicles.

At the end of September, while Jay was picking apples, I flew to England to visit my family. Aunt Joan had deteriorated and was barely lucid, and when I sat beside her bed she called me Brosie, the family's pet name for my mother. It was an easy mistake as we were so alike, but it distressed my father dreadfully. His anguish was visceral and I later found him lying on a bed sobbing that he had burned his Brosie (my mother was cremated). Poor darling, he was all over the place. It was a raw memory that I've carried for ever.

My wonderful aunt Joan died in early November 1978, five years after my mother. Of all the adults in my life when I was growing up, Aunt Joan had been the one who had never laughed at my wild ideas of being a writer. She had encouraged me and bought the best presents – *Roget's Thesaurus*, a typewriter, a writing case, a silver frame for a picture of my grandmother and a seal ring – all of which, except the outmoded typewriter, I can see now from my desk.

Our sojourn in Switzerland came to an abrupt end in February 1979. Jay had been working as a 'pister' on the slopes, which meant keeping the snow smooth under T-bars and pommel lifts, filling in holes on the pistes, helping people who had fallen over and tidying up the mess they had made. At the end of the day, when the ski lifts were closed, pisters skied the runs to ensure that no one was left on the mountain. In the fading light, Jay was halfway home when he hit the side of a bridge. There were no broken bones, but his knee was like a football and he couldn't walk. There was no way he would be skiing for a while.

We decided to travel through Europe, but it's strange how Fate takes a hand. After leaving Greece we moved on to India where we participated in a guaranteed weight-loss programme called amoebic dysentery. Frail but alive, and without much discussion or forward planning, we limped back to Sydney. Somehow, for both of us, Australia felt like home.

We moved into an apartment at Balmoral Beach in Sydney and goofed around for a few years importing Oriental artifacts from India, holidaying in Tahiti and travelling in Australia. We spent another summer in New York and then Jay's parents, Jay and Stella, came to Australia for our southern summer.

By 1982, Jay was teaching full time and the nursing bug was again nipping at my ankles, but what sort of nursing did I want to do? After my five-day brilliant career at Sydney Hospital, and the ongoing media reports of nurses railing against staffing levels and poor conditions in New South Wales hospitals, I wasn't keen on the hospital system. And for certain I was on their DO NOT CALL list.

Advances in medicine and technology, and different ways of delivering health services had opened up new fields of nursing, and I was canvassing further training when an ex-housemate called to say that a letter had arrived for me from the Sydney Opera House Trust.

I broke the land-speed record running round to pick it up.

CHAPTER 26

A Thousand Nights at the Opera

Sydney Opera House, Australia: 1982–9

I HAD LOVED opera, ballet and classical music since childhood, and suddenly I was in the thick of it, employed as a nursing sister in the relief pool at one of the most famous buildings on earth. It was unbelievable and I badly wanted to tell my mother, but that wasn't possible, so I sent postcards of Sydney Opera House to everyone I had ever met. I must have spent my first day's pay on cards and stamps.

Architecturally splendid, with soaring roof shells, Sydney Opera House stands on Bennelong Point in Sydney Harbour, guarding the city like a brilliant white sentinel. Rather dwarfed by the enormity of the adjacent Sydney Harbour Bridge, the building is much larger than it at first appears, and way more than an Opera House. Apart from the Concert Hall (beneath the largest roof shells), the Opera Theatre (beneath the middle roof shells, and now called the Joan Sutherland Theatre) and the restaurant (beneath the smaller roof shells), there is a variety of other performing art spaces.

As a relief sister I was called in when permanent staff were on leave, and there was a lot of work, sometimes weeks at a time. Responsible for the health and safety of staff, performers and patrons, the registered nurse on duty responded to emergency calls throughout the building and grounds, and provided a clinical service in the first-aid room. There were two shifts: 8 a.m. to 4 p.m. and 4 p.m. to midnight, although a nurse remained after hours if companies were 'bumping out', the theatrical term for dismantling a set at the end of a show's run, including removing rigging lights and props. 'Bumping in' was the opposite. Both had attendant risks.

The nurse's workload at Sydney Opera House was a cornucopia of possibilities: a trombone player with an earplug stuck in his ear; a dancer accidentally hit on the mouth by a clarinet; a tourist tumbling down steps; a pregnant woman's waters breaking during *Don Giovanni*; an enormous man suffering chest pain in the Concert Hall; a chef burning his hand in the Bennelong Restaurant; scenery falling on technical staff during a rehearsal in the Drama Theatre; a drunk passing out in the main foyer; a cyclist crashing into a pedestrian on the concourse . . . and the usual colds, headaches and other health problems that ailed staff and performers, who refused to take time off because the show must go on.

During my first week I received an emergency call from the stage door.

'Sister, a thirty-year-old male diver has crawled out of the harbour. He's been hit by a stingray.'

'Where is he?' I asked, my heart quickening. A

busy day, I'd already had half the cast of a Folkloric Festival fainting and vomiting from nerves.

'At Man O'War Steps. A fireman is coming for you.'

Relieved, I put down the phone. There were permanent fire officers at the Opera House and until I knew my way around I was accompanied to all call-outs. It was also routine for a fireman to accompany nurses on call-outs to the auditorium in case a sick patron had to be lifted from the middle of a row.

I was ready with the emergency chair, first-aid bag and resuscitator when the fireman arrived to collect me and we made our way outside.

Man O'War Steps descend into Sydney Harbour on the eastern side of the Opera House, near the Royal Botanic Gardens. The diver was lying near the top of the steps, fully conscious and in obvious agony. Someone had partially rolled up one leg of his wetsuit to form an effective tourniquet above a nasty wound on his calf. Seawater had spread the blood, making it look worse than it probably was.

'I'm Sister from the Opera House,' I said, trying not to sound overly important as people moved aside – there was always the risk of being upstaged by a passing heart surgeon.

Shock from blood loss is the major concern with any wound, and I pulled on gloves and an apron, grabbed a thick dressing pad from the first-aid bag, and gently inspected the injury. Stingrays have venomous serrated spines in their tails, which can break off. I couldn't see any spines protruding, but that didn't mean there wasn't a broken piece inside the man's leg. The wound was about a half-inch wide and, despite the wetsuit tourniquet, was still bleeding.

Placing a small pillow under the diver's head, I checked his vital signs, which were normal, considering the pain. I asked his name, which was Mark, and if he had any pre-existing medical conditions, which he hadn't. He was cold and wet, but had good colour and was breathing easily.

'Did you see the stingray?' I asked. Such a wound could have come from a sharp piece of metal.

Mark nodded. 'I stood on it and the tail whipped up.' He winced in pain. 'I saw it swim away.'

'How long ago?' I asked.

'It just happened. I was about to get out when it hit me.'

The venom, I knew, would already be acting and Mark needed to have the wound properly cleaned in hospital. He would be in pain and feel unwell for a while, and more than likely need antibiotics to prevent wound infection, but he would recover.

'I don't think the barb has hit any important blood vessels,' I said to reassure him, 'but I'll send you to hospital to make sure there isn't anything left in your leg.' I glanced at the fireman, who walked a short distance away and radioed the stage door to telephone for an ambulance and alert Sydney Hospital, which was two minutes up the road.

'Try to stay still, Mark,' I said, covering him with a blanket. Unnecessary movement would force venom through his body. For the same reason I decided not to unzip his wetsuit and ease out an arm to take his blood pressure. I could see he wasn't in shock, but to be on the safe side I prepared the resuscitator and placed scissors nearby in case I had to quickly cut his wetsuit.

'You're doing fine,' I said, as I poured normal saline over the wound to clean out some of the debris. I was loath to release the tourniquet and apply pressure for fear of forcing any broken barb further into his leg.

Mark was already having muscle cramps in both legs from the venom when the paramedics arrived. We swapped blankets and pillows and they took his details, eased him out of the top part of his wetsuit, assessed his vital signs, established an IV and cut the leg of his wetsuit to release the tourniquet. It appeared the bleeding had stopped.

'Were you diving alone?' one paramedic asked, and I grimaced. I should have asked that.

'Yes, it's stupid, I know,' Mark said.

'We'll run you up to Sydney Hospital, mate,' the paramedic said. 'Let the docs have a look at you.'

Bagging my used gloves and apron, I watched them load Mark into the ambulance and drive away. 'Don't mention you know me when you get to Sydney Hospital!' I called out softly.

Back in the first-aid room, I completed an accident form and that was when I realized I hadn't asked for a phone number to contact someone on Mark's behalf. Apparently, it would take a few emergencies for me to have all my ducks in a row.

After replenishing the first-aid bag, I checked my pager was on and returned to the steps with a bucket of water to wash away any spilled blood. You see, Mark had pulled himself ashore at a significant military spot. Man O'War Steps had been the embarkation point for sailors who had left Australia to serve in the First World War, the Second World War, Korea, Malaya and Vietnam, and more than two thousand of them had never returned.

Daily rounds of the building were an important part of the nurse's routine at Sydney Opera House. It allowed us to identify potential hazards, assess the wellbeing of staff who were returning to work after an illness, and monitor the emergency medical equipment that was hidden in secret cupboards behind the wooden panelling of the building's interior. This could easily take a couple of hours, especially if I had to double back to the first-aid room for a hot water bottle to ease a conductor's rheumatic back.

The first-aid room was located off the Green Room, where performers, company crew and house staff relaxed and had refreshments. There was a two-bed area that could be curtained off, the main clinical room with the nurse's desk and medical equipment, another smaller space, which could also be curtained off, and a bathroom where I spruced myself up if I'd been sailing before my shift and then dropped off at Man O'War Steps.

Some days the first-aid room was hectic – a trumpeter holding an ice pack on his lips, a patron resting on one bed after falling over, and an actor with a migraine on the other. At other times I might not see a soul in the first-aid room all day. But you never knew what was around the corner.

One evening I was called to the Ladies near the box office. A large American woman from a visiting cruise ship had collapsed, luckily not behind a locked door. It was a warm evening and she was weighed down with diamonds and a heavy fur coat, which, at that time, you could still wear without attracting criticism – though I thought it had probably looked much better on its original owner. She was dazed and sitting on the floor like a deflated grizzly bear when I arrived.

My initial assessment was that she had fainted.

'May I help?' asked a well-dressed woman. 'I'm a doctor.'

'A medical doctor?' I asked. Lately, everyone with an academic qualification was calling themselves a doctor.

She smiled. 'Yes, a GP.'

As you can imagine, there was always a doctor at the Opera House somewhere, and I appreciated their offer to help, particularly if someone was having a coronary during a performance inside the Opera Theatre or Concert Hall. As long as they showed medical ID and I recorded their details, I handed them the bag of tricks.

It wasn't unusual, I told the doctor as she examined the woman, for passengers from cruise ships to hurry an evening meal, put on heavy coats, then rush to the performance and pass out. Mrs Melvyn Jackson from St Augustine, Florida, confirmed that that was exactly what she had done.

'You need a short rest and a glass of water,' the doctor declared, as we settled Mrs Jackson in the emergency chair. I thanked the doctor and an usher escorted her to the Opera Theatre as *Così fan tutte* had already started. I rounded up Mr Jackson, who was outside wondering where his wife had gone, and took both Americans to the first-aid room.

'Melvyn, will you look at this!' Mrs Jackson exclaimed. 'It's like a small hospital!'

I helped her on to a bed, checked her over again, fetched iced water from the Green Room and pulled a chair next to the bed for Mr Jackson.

'What did you have tickets for?' I asked.

'The opera,' Mrs Jackson said. She turned to her husband. 'Oh, Melvyn, I'm sorry. I know how much you wanted to see the show.'

'It can't be helped,' Melvyn said, failing miserably to hide his disappointment.

'Watch this,' I said, and turned on the television at the foot of her bed, then switched the dial until I found the channel designated for the Opera Theatre. 'It's in black and white, I'm afraid, but you can watch the first act here and, if you feel well enough, I'll have someone show you to your seats during the intermission.'

Mrs Jackson grabbed her husband's hand. 'How wonderful is this, Melvyn?'

Melvyn smiled profusely. 'They'll never believe it back home, Thelma.'

By the intermission Mrs Jackson was fine and ready to be taken to the Opera Theatre.

'Pay the nurse, will you, Melvyn?' she ordered.

'There's no charge,' I said.

Mrs Jackson turned to her husband. 'My, oh my, is this a great country or what, Melvyn?'

On quiet evenings I recorded cassette tapes of news for my father, who was married to the third Mrs Johnson, a woman I had never met. They had sold their lovely old house in West Liss and moved to Dorset, where my long-retired father had taken up a job as a night-watchman at Poole Yacht Club – a pastime that was short-lived when there was a shoot-out one night between drug dealers and police. Herbie J had then bought a motorbike and leather riding gear and, according to my sister-in-law Esther, was currently terrorizing the upmarket neighbourhood where they were living.

Thanking me for the tapes, my father sent cards in which he put photographs and the words *letter to follow*. I rarely received the letter to follow, but from the ones I did, I gathered my father was spending a lot of time with my brother's family, who were living in Dibden Purlieu, near the New Forest. Ben had a small catamaran called *Herbie J* and grandfather and grandson were messing about together in sheds and on boats. It was good to hear.

It was incredibly humbling and at the same time immensely thrilling to be in the presence of amazing talent. It pierced all my defences and turned me into a bumbling idiot who could lose the power of speech. Perhaps the most instantly recognizable performer who literally glowed with out-of-this-galaxy incandescence was the Italian tenor Luciano Pavarotti. He was in the box office foyer when I first saw him offstage, I think signing copies of his book, *My Own Story*. He had the turning circle of the *Queen Mary*, so the term *larger than life* might have been coined especially for him, and it would have made a much better book title. I sensed that he was trying to look like a regular guy, but he couldn't pull it off. Pavarotti's luminescent smile lit up his whole face and it was difficult not to genuflect and walk backwards away from him.

There were also times when I didn't recognize famous performers, which was a profound embarrassment and made me want to crawl into a hole. Also, I continually mistook the maestros in their penguin suits – the conductors who, let's face it, the majority of us only ever see from behind.

But let's return to my mistakes. One quiet evening I was watching a play on the television in the first-aid room when a woman popped her head around the door and asked, 'Have you got a minute, Sister? I've something in my eye and I daren't poke at it with my stage make-up on.'

'Please, come in,' I said, recognizing the famous soprano immediately. Trying not to appear flustered in her presence, I sat down, switched on the light and carefully teased out an offending eyelash.

'There, that's got it,' I said proudly. 'I'll just note your details in the day book.'

And that was when my mind went blank. No way could I recall her name. Sensing my quandary, she prompted, 'It's Joan.'

'Of course,' I said, and carefully wrote 'Joan Sutherland' in elaborate cursive script so she could comment on my artistic handwriting.

'Actually, I'm the other Joan – Joan Carden,' she said, with absolutely no trace of the outraged self-regard that she was entitled to. Smiling sweetly, she patted my hand. 'But not to worry, it happens all the time.'

Real class. In spades.

CHAPTER 27

Misadventures in Paradise

Great Barrier Reef, Australia: 1983–4

HIDDEN IN THE back pages of the newspaper was an advertisement seeking a registered nurse for the resort at South Molle, one of the idyllic islands scattered amongst the fringing reefs and coral shoals in the heart of the Great Barrier Reef Marine Park. Images of lofty peaks, blue bays and sugar-white sandy beaches floated in front of my eyes, for Jay and I had been there before and knew it was paradise.

In disbelief I read the ad again, but it was real, all right, and it was a dream job. My hands trembled with excitement as I dialled the long-distance phone number from Sydney to North Queensland.

'Hold the line,' a disembodied voice ordered.

Then there was a long silence. I was about to disconnect when a woman said, 'Are you calling about the nursing position?'

'Yes,' I said, and braced myself for her to say that the job had gone. But she didn't and, after a multitude of questions, the position was mine if my references checked out.

'The nurse holds a one-hour surgery five afternoons

321

a week,' she explained, 'and for the rest of your work hours, you'll be serving in the gift shop while on call.' Wages, she added, would reflect both positions and I would have two days off a week.

'Who will cover the nurse position on my days off?' I asked. Free time in paradise needed to be free.

'Another staff member who is an RN.'

On a roll, I asked about work for Jay.

'What can he do?'

'Oh, anything,' I answered boldly.

'Are you married?' she asked, a hint of exasperation in her voice.

The relevance of this made me pause before answering that, yes, we were married. Otherwise I surmised she might not bother finding Jay a position.

'Hold the line,' she said, and I heard footsteps walking away.

In fact, Jay and I had been married for five months. As per my grand plan, I was thirty years old, and the wedding had been a stress-free, no-frills register-office ceremony celebrated with friends in Sydney, the groom still wearing golf clothes from an earlier game and the bride looking fabulous in a burgundy gypsy skirt and peasant blouse. We hadn't bothered with an engagement, or told our respective families overseas until after the event. To their credit, both families had made a good show of regretting that they hadn't attended the nuptials, but I think they were secretly relieved. For them, Australia was the end of the known world in travel terms.

I heard footsteps again and the phone was picked up.

'There's a gardening position,' she offered.

'Oh, Jay loves gardening!' I lied enthusiastically.

*

'What the heck' has always been a good decision-making tool for Jay and me, and it was two days after Christmas when we landed with two suitcases and Jay's windsurfer at a hot and humid Proserpine airport to the north of the Tropic of Capricorn on the Queensland coast. Wilting from the intense heat and steaming humidity, we caught the local bus to Shute Harbour and boarded the *Island Wanderer* to take us out through the sapphire waters of the Whitsunday Passage to our new home.

The resort on South Molle was marketed as relaxed and informal, which we assumed was a fancy way of saying that things were not being upgraded. It occupied only a small part of the island, the rest being roughly two thousand acres of national park, with no roads or cars. When we had stayed as guests, the slightly shabby edges hadn't mattered as it had been the natural beauty of the island that had won our hearts. That, plus the availability of every sport imaginable – golf, tennis, squash, kayaking, windsurfing, water-skiing, swimming, snorkelling, diving, sailing and hiking the wonderful trails.

We checked in as staff, so there were no friendly greetings before a stern-faced woman with skin like a crocodile's handed us a pile of bedding. Looking at the red hibiscus flower that Jay had picked and put in my hair, she remarked that picking flowers was forbidden and failure to comply with rules was instant dismissal. 'It's called being NBO'd,' she said, seemingly proud of knowing something we didn't. 'It stands for Next Boat Out.'

'Thanks for telling us,' I said, and defiantly left the flower in my hair as I signed for the bedding. Frowning, she pointed us on our way and we lugged our gear to the staff quarters behind a fence at the rear of the resort. Beyond the bathrooms and staff bar, accommodation was provided in randomly placed cheap cabins, old caravans propped between palm trees, and rows of small shed-like structures called dongas. It was boggy underfoot from recent tropical rain and there was a pungent odour from fruit left rotting on the ground. Every so often a waft of marijuana floated past us on the breeze.

Our married quarters were a donga furnished with a damp double bed and a chest of drawers that smelt like low tide. The room had the warmth and charm of a Spanish public toilet, but that wasn't the worst part. Sitting on the bed was the world's largest living cane toad. Remembering that the ugly critters had poisonous glands behind their heads, I removed my shoe and slammed it on the mattress. The toad jumped off the bed and, assisted by Jay's toe, rocketed out of the door.

'Well,' I said confidently, 'the room is awful, but it's nothing a spring clean won't fix.'

Jay laughed. 'It's going to need all four seasons,' he said, and I laughed too because it didn't matter. Unlike at other resorts, South Molle staff could mix with guests and use the sports and entertainment facilities when off duty. The state of our room wasn't important.

I'd brought nurse uniforms with me, but was told that advertising medical assistance wasn't appropriate on a holiday island. That seemed reasonable and I was soon outfitted in a blue cotton dress covered with white shell and coral motifs. And I was lucky. Jay had to wear a loose blue-and-white floral shirt and pale blue shorts that made him look like an extra on *Hawaii Five-O*.

We had been on the island only a few days when the first medical drama occurred. I could hear the commotion coming from the beach as I grabbed the nurse's bag of tricks from the first-aid room. Walking fast, I followed Martin, the barman who had fetched me, down to the beach. I would be no use if I ran and arrived out of breath.

A crowd of tourists had gathered around a twenty-something girl in a red bikini who was hopping around and screaming hysterically. There was a mess of blood under her left ankle, but absolutely nothing wrong with her lungs, which any nurse will tell you is a good sign.

Tourists in Australia often fear they will die from whatever physical misfortune has befallen them – vast distances from medical aid and true stories of the most venomous creatures on earth don't help the situation. I grasped the girl's hands and said loudly, 'I'm the island nurse. Calm down.' But she shook free and carried on screaming.

'Stop it!' I shouted in her face.

Suddenly Martin jabbed her in the back of both knees and she dropped to the ground like a sack of sand and stopped screaming. Wide-eyed, she asked, 'Am I going to die?'

'Not on my watch,' I said, and knelt down to inspect her foot.

'What's your name?' I asked.

'Na-Nadia,' she stammered. 'Oh, God, it hurts . . .'

Working quickly, I poured saline over her foot to clear away sand and blood. There were two shallow different-sized wounds about an inch apart in the soft flesh below her ankle. I couldn't see any debris and applied light pressure with a gauze pad to stem the bleeding.

'It's a snake bite,' a male bystander said unhelpfully. 'Two holes like that, it's gotta be a sea snake.'

The bystander was Mr Truscott. I remembered him from the gift shop where he had hired golf clubs and made a song and dance about leaving a deposit.

Nadia's bottom lip trembled. 'It could have been a sea snake,' she whimpered.

'Bites from sea snakes don't hurt,' I told her firmly, 'and they have small, even-sized fangs. These wounds are too big. Besides, I've never heard of anyone dying from a sea-snake bite in Australian waters.' This was true, I hadn't, but that didn't make it fact, although it calmed Nadia.

'Did she see a snake?' Mr Truscott said. 'I bet she saw a snake.'

Biting my tongue, I flashed him the death stare. Turning back to Nadia, I asked, 'Did it happen in the sea?'

Nadia nodded and a tear rolled down her cheek.

'She needs a proper nurse or doctor, not a shop girl,' Mr Truscott said rudely. 'Someone should go to Reception and ask if there's one here.'

It was unbelievable. All my working life I'd been told I looked like a nurse, and now, when I needed to, I looked like a shop girl! I must have grown out of whatever the giveaway nurse signs were. And Truscott was making me realize something else – that a nurse uniform commands respect. Our uniforms of old – those wonderful waisted dresses with detachable collars and cuffs, starched white aprons, wide belts with silver buckles, black stockings, shiny badges and elaborate white bonnets – had commanded more respect from patients and the general public than any nurse uniform had since (except on Dickens ward where only a firearm would have helped).

'Please, Mr Truscott,' I said politely. 'I am a proper nurse.'

Holding his hands up, he backed away. 'She needs help is all I'm saying.'

The bleeding slowed to a trickle and I ran through the possibilities – stonefish, coral cuts, small shark, cone shell, stingray, toadfish – but the skin around her ankle wasn't red or swollen, and it looked more like she'd been pinched by something. Ha! In a flash I realized where I had seen similar wounds before: on my own foot in Tahiti.

Smiling at Nadia, I said, 'You're going to be fine. I'll take you to the first-aid room and dress your foot.'

Fifteen minutes later, cleaned and bandaged, Nadia asked me, 'Do we have to tell people I was pinched by a crab?' I knew she was upset about the drama on the beach.

'It must have been a big crab,' I said supportively.

'I know, but I'm . . .well, I'm embarrassed about screaming the place down.'

I thought for a moment. 'We can say you were attacked by an *amuse-bouche* if you like?'

'That sounds French,' Nadia said, 'like *bêche-de-mer*.'

'It is. It's a small bite of something, in this case you.'

Nadia smiled. 'Yes, I was attacked by an *amuse-bouche*. I like that.'

Jay disliked working in the tropical gardens and the gardens knew it and got even. At the end of each day he was scratched and covered with bug bites. Close to performing cosmetic surgery on the oleanders with a chain saw, he was mercifully plucked from the shrubbery and deposited in the staff bar where, as sole barman, he was placed in charge of alcohol sales and making small-talk with off-duty colleagues. It was a tough gig for somebody, and Jay was that somebody.

As the island nurse I worked under the supervision of the splendid Dr John Parker, whose practice was at Airlie Beach on the mainland. John visited the island for a couple of afternoon surgeries a week and the rest of the time, if necessary, we communicated by telephone.

The small first-aid room was behind the shop and comprised a desk, two chairs, a bed, a fridge and a sink. Shelves and a cupboard held dressings, instruments, medical equipment, a resuscitator and oxygen cylinder. There was a useful array of lotions, ointments and common medications, while dangerous drugs were locked in the manager's office.

A day book recorded patient details and treatment, and there was a file containing phone numbers, accident forms, images of wounds from marine creatures and the identifying sting marks of several types of jellyfish, which I would come to know off by heart. At the time we used vinegar on all jellyfish stings to neutralize the venom, and plunged feet stung by stonefish into hot water, as hot as the patient could take it, to ease the horrific pain.

Mercurochrome was my go-to treatment on wounds for anything to do with oysters, rocks and coral. Warm tropical seawater was adept at causing infection in open cuts and completely hopeless at healing them – unlike the cold grey Atlantic, which dried up and healed sores in a trice. Anyone with an injury that needed an X-ray or difficult suturing was packed off to the mainland on the regular island boat service, and for serious illness and accidents I commandeered the fastest boat available and met the ambulance at Shute Harbour.

Afternoon surgery was always packed. In addition to around five hundred guests, there were about seventy staff employed between the resort and the boats, and on island feast nights the population could swell to almost eight hundred. With so many people, there was always someone needing attention.

It was a dark and stormy night – no, really, it was a dark and stormy night – when Ned, one of the boat skippers, banged on our door at 2 a.m. Most of the marine crew lived on the mainland with their families, but Ned and Mack, a deckhand, had stayed on the island after the previous night's sunset cruise was cancelled due to bad weather.

'Maggie,' Ned yelled over the rain, 'Mack's sick!'

'Coming,' I called sleepily, forced myself out of bed and dressed. I knew Mack had a stomach ulcer and that he was under doctor's orders to eat regular meals and refrain from booze. At the time it was believed peptic ulcers were hereditary and caused by stress and occupations with irregular mealtimes.

Outside, Ned was sitting on our veranda, soaked from the rain. Sharing an umbrella, we sloshed through the mud to the cabin where Mack and he were staying. Poor Mack was doubled up with stomach pain. There was blood in the vomit in the bucket beside the bed.

He was cold and clammy to touch and his pulse was rapid.

'I'm so cold,' Mack wailed.

Covering him with another blanket, I asked when the vomiting had started.

'About half an hour ago.'

'Is the pain worse than last time?'

'Christ, yes, it's burning,' Mack managed.

I felt his abdomen. It was hard and distended. I didn't like the look of this and feared the ulcer had perforated the lining of his stomach. He could be haemorrhaging. 'Is it possible to take a boat over to Shute Harbour in this weather?' I asked Ned. 'Mack needs to be hospitalized.'

'It'll be rough,' Ned said, 'but we can do it if we have to.'

'Stay with Mack,' I told him, and raced to the nearest phone. It was 3 a.m. and I called Proserpine Hospital on the mainland and spoke to a doctor in the emergency room. He told me to put up a normal saline IV and give Mack morphine for the pain. 'Can you bring a boat across in this storm?' he asked.

'Apparently,' I told him.

'I'll organize an ambulance to meet you at Shute Harbour.' He rattled off his radio wavelength so I could talk to him from the boat.

While Ned and other helpers who had woken up loaded Mack on to the flat-bed truck that we used to cart things around the resort, I ran to the first-aid room and gathered things I would need. I had to wake a duty manager to access the morphine, then check the dose with the hospital and record it before giving the drug to Mack, which took more time than I wanted.

It would take ages to reach Shute Harbour in these conditions and I stupidly decided to put the IV up on the boat. I hadn't put up an IV since Switzerland, but at least I knew how to do it. On a ward. On solid ground.

It was a nightmare ride over to the mainland. The storm was chucking all it had at us – huge waves, wind and rain – but somehow, in the roll and pitch of the boat, I put up the IV. A lucky lurch of the boat found Mack's vein, although I took full credit.

Mack's pain had eased but he was still retching when our boat thumped against the jetty at Shute Harbour. The paramedics took over and Mack was hurried to Proserpine Hospital where he received a blood transfusion, the bleeding stopped and he was hospitalized for rest. Two weeks later he was a mended man and returned to work. Thanks to Mack, Jay and I never paid for another trip to the outer reef or other islands for the rest of our time in the Whitsundays. Needless to say, we took full advantage of this, bought disposable underwater cameras and snorkelled the hell out of the reef.

June to August were winter months on the reef. Temperatures eased, tourist numbers diminished and considerable numbers of staff were NBO'd, I imagine to reduce costs. Not wanting to be casualties of the cuts, we decided to visit family and friends in England and America, then return to South Molle Island in a few months. I also wanted to work a few days at Sydney Opera House – I needed to put in at least one day every six months to maintain my position in the relief pool.

Financially, we were okay. While some staff were drinking their own weight in rum before passing out, Jay and I had been taking advantage of the island's free amenities and banking our salaries. With a few whimpers, Jay sold his windsurfer (in case we didn't return) and we flew to Sydney for a week before heading overseas for the northern hemisphere summer.

In September, we returned to South Molle Island. The trade winds were still hammering the resort and we had an immediate sense that something on the island wasn't right. Rumours were rife. There were stories of a peeping Tom in the staff quarters and that the resort owners were in financial trouble, and I have to say there were a lot of glum faces about. More of our work colleagues were being NBO'd, and we shortly received a letter from the Queensland branch of the Australian Workers' Union, advising us that they had received complaints from staff leaving the island that threats had been made to them if they contacted the union. This shocked and surprised us, as we had become friendly with a couple of the young duty managers and we knew they would not countenance such behaviour.

In time there were problems with the island water supply, and remaining staff, including ourselves, were reduced to a four-day week.

'What do you think about leaving?' Jay asked me one evening.

'I think it's a good idea,' I said.

But we weren't quick enough. A few days later Jay and I were NBO'd. And we didn't care because it was a point of honour to be NBO'd from South Molle Island.

We had lived the island's golden age, and it was hard to imagine it would ever be as good again.

In December we returned to Sydney and moved into a house-sit two doors up from Bambi and Rod at Balmoral Beach. It was good to be with friends again, and a novelty to embrace the real world of driving, shopping and cooking. Plus it was an absolute joy to be near a library.

Jay contacted the New South Wales Department of Education and requested a mathematics position in Sydney, and I returned to casual work at Sydney Opera House. Jay was quickly offered teaching posts in Sydney that nobody else wanted, which he just as quickly refused. By way of punishment he was offered a position at a central school in a remote Australian town called Wee Waa (pronounced we war) – central schools were established in rural and isolated Australian communities to provide education for both primary and high-school students. To most people, Wee Waa was in the back of beyond, but to us it was where friends of ours lived on their cotton farms.

Deciding that it might be a good experience to work in the bush for a while, and fantastic to spend more time with our rural friends, we took a chance and went to Wee Waa.

CHAPTER 28

Two in the Bush

Wee Waa, New South Wales: 1985

THE SMALL OUTBACK town of Wee Waa sits under the vast open skies of the north-west plains of New South Wales. Summer days are hot, winter nights are cold, and the vagaries of precipitation deliver anything from drought to overflowing creeks.

About three hundred and sixty miles from Sydney, Wee Waa is famously known as the cotton capital of Australia. Surrounded by rich agricultural soil, in addition to growing tons of wheat and grazing squillions of sheep for wool, the land produces oceans of fabulous cotton.

Of course, coming from England I'd seen sheep and wheat before; just never quite so many sheep and a field of wheat the size of Shropshire. The first time I saw cotton, I was amazed; it truly was cotton wool balls growing on a small bush. And there was so much of it – an endless horizon of white fluffy land dotted with farm machinery the size of suburban bungalows. Even some of the cockies (farmers) were six foot twenty.

A week after Jay started teaching at Wee Waa

Central School, I was employed as the Aboriginal health nurse at the community health centre in Rose Street, the wide, straight road in the middle of town.

My job was not identified, which meant I did not have to be Aboriginal to hold the position, but that of the Aboriginal health worker was identified, and it was held by Denise, a bubbly young woman with a spectacular singing voice. Denise was my passport into her complex and ancient culture and its connections with the land and nature, so different from my own cultural heritage, which had been forged almost entirely by man-made constructs and global history.

Our mandate at the community health centre was to assist rural families to enjoy good health and negotiate their access to medical and social services, many of which were some distance away. My specific task as the Aboriginal health nurse was to address the health and social issues of the most marginalized and disadvantaged in the community, which was assumed to be the Aboriginal population, but there were marginalized and disadvantaged white folk too. Oppressive poverty, overcrowded living conditions, alcoholism, gambling, nutritional problems, drug addiction and rotten luck didn't discriminate.

Throughout Australia, parcels of land called missions or reserves had been set aside for Indigenous Aboriginals to live on. The missions were controlled by churches, and the reserves were under the auspices of whatever government was in power and the Aboriginal Land Council. The Pines was a large reserve outside Wee Waa where Denise and I visited many Aboriginal families. A mixture of scrub and semi-arid woodland of cypress pine and eucalypt trees, there was no formal structure to the place. An attempt had been made to build a few brick houses, but they had been gutted and the wooden window frames and doors used for firewood. There was also an abandoned pig farm with sties, but no pigs.

The residents lived in shacks they had built themselves out of wood, sticks, canvas, discarded doors, sheets of corrugated iron and tarpaulins. As a nod to modern conveniences, there was an ablutions block with no lavatory seats or doors, no toilet paper and only cold running water. Lately, for a reason that I never established, someone had been removing the shower rose, so each trip out I replaced it with a new one. Heaven knows what the man at the hardware store thought I was doing with them all, but my mother would have been pleased to see me still wielding a wrench as part of my nursing role.

It was mid-autumn and cold when I drove out to The Pines to check on a young boy I had seen from a distance on a few previous visits, and who never seemed to be at school. I parked near a shack beneath a massive she-oak from where I could see him playing with a toy truck in the dirt. Rather skinny, he looked about seven years old. I got out of the car and walked towards him. Closer inspection revealed the boy's nose caked in dried green snot and muck leaking from his ears.

'Hello,' I said. 'My name's Maggie. What's yours?'

'That's Alfie,' an older Aboriginal woman answered for him. 'He can't hear ya, and he can't speak neither.'

'What, never?' I questioned.

Barefoot and wearing a voluminous red skirt and a

black jumper, she was sitting on a plastic chair and whittling a stick with a penknife. Her mass of unruly grey hair was piled on top of her head and tied with a brown shoelace.

She shook her head. 'Deaf and dumb,' she said. 'So he stops with me. Alfie's me grandson.'

'May I sit down?' I asked, indicating another plastic chair.

'Yeah,' she said. 'And don't break it. We have a lot of trouble with your lot breaking our things.'

'I'll try not to,' I said, and sat down to watch Alfie for a while. He was wearing jeans and a blue sweatshirt and appeared perfectly content pushing the truck through the dirt.

'Is Alfie's mother around?' I asked at length.

'Out Walgett way,' the woman said. 'With her new bloke.'

'Well, is the old bloke around?'

'He's in Silverwater.'

Silverwater was a prison in Sydney. I let an appropriate amount of time pass before asking, 'Has Alfie seen a doctor? He might have an ear infection.'

Hearing loss was a serious issue in the bush, not only for farmers and labourers who worked with noisy farm machinery, but also for Aboriginal youngsters with chronic ear infections that hadn't been treated because of remote living conditions. These children were prone to glue ear, where the middle ear filled with a sticky glue-like fluid that interrupted sound vibrations and caused hearing loss. Without treatment, glue ear inevitably led to poor speech development and educational difficulties. I suspected this might be the problem with Alfie.

But the woman shook her head and I wasn't surprised. There was much suspicion and distrust of authority and whitefella ways among the indigenous population.

'How about I make an appointment with a doctor to treat Alfie's nose and ears, and I'll do a hearing test?' I said. 'I'll come and collect you and bring you both back here afterwards.'

She looked suspicious. 'Both of us? Back here?'

'Of course both of you. What else would I do?'

'I'll think about it,' she said, and went back to whittling, which I gathered meant she'd had enough of me.

The following morning I made a doctor's appointment for Alfie and drove out to The Pines to pass on the information. But Alfie and his grandmother were gone. I asked another woman if she knew where they were or when they'd be back.

'They're not coming back,' she said. 'In case you take Alfie away.'

I was stunned. 'Why would I do that?'

The woman shrugged. 'Cos that's what you people do.'

At the health centre, in addition to treating an occasional pet lamb for ringworm, we conducted hearing tests and ran clinics for diabetes, high blood pressure, drug and alcohol counselling, family planning and diet, and to combat the poor uptake of immunizations we travelled to outlying villages to immunize babies and children.

A couple of times a week, we had meetings with the director of nursing at Wee Waa Hospital, the small community facility that provided emergency and general medical care for residents of Wee Waa and the surrounding district. Overseen by a local GP, registered nurses managed the day-to-day care at the hospital and everything ticked along nicely.

Recovery from illness was difficult for anyone living rough, and after our meetings I visited Aboriginal clients who were hospitalized, sometimes for relatively minor illnesses. A bad cold could easily become pneumonia if you slept under the stars, and influenza could be fatal without proper care. Mothers with sick children tried their best, but without access to clean water, a bed or a roof over their heads, the youngsters were vulnerable to complications from normal childhood diseases. For those families, Wee Waa Hospital and the wonderful nurses were a godsend, and I was especially touched by the night nurses, who knitted jumpers for the children to keep them warm when they went home.

After patients were discharged from hospital, I made follow-up visits to change dressings, test blood pressure, blood sugar, and check medications. These home visits could be in town or conducted in the bush beside the work car, while batting away flies. Both the car and I wore a skirt of red dust from the dirt roads and I could be wet as well if I had stood in the creek with a mother and helped her treat a child's head lice.

Honestly, I have no idea how some of the families coped with the conditions and situations they had to live with. Can you imagine not having a birth certificate? But it was a fact of life for many Aboriginal people born in outback camps, on reserves and missions, or elsewhere in the bush. This made access to support pensions difficult as there were no birth records, they had no bank accounts, and many had no income at all, relying on those who did and local charities. Poverty, I learned, was a cruel mistress, and as Denise and I helped illiterate and desperate folk to jump bureaucratic hurdles, judgement by the fortunate and well-fed was an ever-present issue.

Slowly Jay and I were fitting in to the social fabric of Wee Waa and enjoying working and living in the bush. Jay joined the baseball team and played golf at the local course where kangaroos watched him putt on sand greens, and I spent much of my free time writing short stories that I sent to magazine editors who didn't bother replying. I also joined a pottery class and produced a range of lumpy mugs and solid vases. Nobody wanted those either.

We had good times with our friends but I always had a sense that it all wasn't quite right. Since we'd arrived in Wee Waa, I'd had a feeling that something important was missing, but I couldn't work out what it was. It would come to me, I thought.

Spring was drifting in when Jay was offered a teaching position at an academic private school in Sydney. It was tempting for several reasons. We had saved the deposit to buy an apartment, it was a good time to enter the Sydney housing market, and banks were giving mortgages to anyone nuts enough to pay fifteen per cent interest. And I was pretty sure that if Jay didn't own another sailboat soon he would spontaneously combust. I'd also realized what the important something was that had been missing since we had arrived in Wee Waa. It was the sea.

Living and working in the bush had been a great

experience, but here was a chance for a new adventure. We dithered over a decision for five minutes until one of us said, 'Oh, what the heck!'

With hugs and emotional goodbyes, we rode out of town.

Not long after our return to Sydney in 1985, we purchased a small garden apartment near the harbour and a part share in a yacht. Jay was teaching and I began work as a community nurse specialist, organizing equipment and appliances for people with disabilities. I worked nine days every two weeks, so there was ample time to continue my casual position at Sydney Opera House, not only for free tickets but to maintain my practical nursing skills. I was still busily penning short stories in the evenings, on days off and during quiet times at the Opera House.

With employer approval I worked both positions until 1989 when I took maternity leave from the disability position. Hopelessly stage-struck, I continued working at Sydney Opera House until my tummy was so big that I couldn't squeeze between rows of seats without suffocating members of the audience.

My last day of nursing was at Sydney Opera House. It was a fitting way to mark the finale of a much-loved career and the opening act of my new life as a mother and struggling writer. Who knew if I'd be successful at the writing part? Jay, in his usual pragmatic way, said that being successful wasn't important – it was having a go that mattered. So I planned to keep on having a go at writing while our baby slept for those long hours they are supposed to, and you can imagine how well that worked out for me.

The skills I'd learned as a nurse came in handy. Nursing had taught me to physically multitask while thinking about something else, to walk fast, function on little sleep, look calm when I wasn't, hang on for hours with a full bladder, and to question explanations that I didn't understand. It had shown me that hope was the most powerful of all emotions, that working at something I enjoyed was more important than making money, that sensitivity was a strength, that the touch of a human hand was everything to the sick and the frightened, and that giving was more rewarding than receiving.

Perhaps the most valuable lesson I learned was that men and women, when they grow old and frail, seem to regret the things that they hadn't done when they were young and had the chance – and I can honestly say that I heard that message loud and clear in the early months of my training. From then on I walked through every door that opened for me.

Along the way, in addition to gathering a startling collection of funny, sad, troubling, touching and occasionally shocking stories, I made wonderful lifelong friends and experienced the delights and disappointments, the joys and sadness, and the thrills and spills of an amazing nursing career. And I loved every scary, rewarding, back-breaking minute.

I'd do it all again in a heartbeat.

Thanks

NOT YOUR AVERAGE *Nurse* was originally written for my daughter, Hannah, and it is an account of my nursing career before she was born and grew up knowing me as a struggling writer. The catalyst was the bitter regret that I had known so little of my own mother's working life, and I wanted to redress any lack of maternal hand-me-down work experience for Hannah. I also needed her to understand that I haven't always been the boring one in the study with her elbow on the desk and a faraway look in her eyes.

Huge thanks to my husband, Jay, for his endless belief in me, and I owe a sincere debt of gratitude to my friend and literary agent Selwa Anthony who, for almost twenty years, has been my guiding light in the literary world. Thanks too, to Brian Dennis, Linda Anthony and Drew Keys for their hard work on my behalf. Team Anthony rules.

On the nursing side of things, I have not been alone in summoning memories. For their enduring friendship and assistance delving into the past, I send heartfelt thanks to Gillian Cooper, Bernice Forsyth, Bambi Hanson, Kathy Lee and Jan Turner. Thanks also to Judy and Peter Donald for providing their sunroom for occasional writing purposes, and to Sandie and Nick Helyer for tracking down a much-needed resource.

Bringing a book to life takes many people. In Australia, thanks must go to Sophie Ambrose, Commissioning Editor at Penguin Random House Australia, for her patience, professional guidance and expertly nurturing this book and its author through the editorial and publishing process, and to Kevin O'Brien and Pamela Dunne for their fine editorial skills. In the United Kingdom, thanks must go to Andrea Henry, Editorial Director at Transworld Publishers, Penguin Random House UK, for her professional guidance, encouraging words and publishing expertise, to Helena Gonda for her editorial assistance, and to Hazel Orme who polished every page.

I couldn't have done it alone.

Maggie Groff
Nelson Bay